Dr Mark Weatherall is a Consultant Neurologist and Clinical Lead for Neurology at Buckinghamshire Healthcare NHS Trust, former Chair of the British Association for the Study of Headache and Trustee of The Migraine Trust. He was a highly regarded historian of medicine before studying clinical medicine at Cambridge. Junior medical jobs followed in Cambridge, London and Oxford, before he completed his specialist training in neurology in the North-West of England. He spent twelve months as a clinical research fellow at the Institute of Neurology in London. He is a Fellow of the Royal Colleges of Physicians of London and Edinburgh.

His interests include the diagnosis and management of chronic migraine, facial pain, visual snow and secondary headaches associated with systemic disorders, as well as the historical, social and cultural aspects of headache disorders. He has made presentations on these subjects at recent meetings of the International Headache Society, the European Headache Federation, the Migraine Trust International Symposium and the Association of British Neurologists. He actively promotes the importance of headache disorders through social media such as X, formerly known as Twitter (@weatherallmw) and more traditional media platforms.

T0349323

Living with Headaches

DR MARK WEATHERALL

Copyright © Dr Mark Weatherall

The right of Dr Mark Weatherall to be identified as the Author of the Work has been asserted by him in accordance with the Copyright, Designs and Patents Act 1988.

First published in paperback in 2024 by Headline Home an imprint of Headline Publishing Group

2

Cataloguing in Publication Data is available from the British Library

Paperback ISBN 978 1 4722 9830 0
e-ISBN 978 1 4722 9831 7

Typeset in Dante by CC Book Production
Printed and bound in Great Britain by Clays Ltd, Elcograf S.p.A.

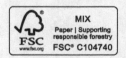

MIX
Paper | Supporting
responsible forestry
FSC® C104740

HEADLINE PUBLISHING GROUP
An Hachette UK Company
Carmelite House
50 Victoria Embankment
London
EC4Y 0DZ

www.headline.co.uk
www.hachette.co.uk

For my patients, past, present and future

Contents

Introduction   1

The Basics

What is a headache?   3

What type of headache do I have?   6

Common primary headaches   9

Common secondary headaches   14

What causes chronic headaches   18

When does having headaches become an illness?   22

The Science Bit

Where does the pain of headache come from?   29

What is CGRP, and what does it have to do
    with headache?   35

What is aura?   41

What are the varieties of visual aura?   46

What other types of aura are there?   50

What causes aura?   59

Treatments: acute, preventive and lifestyle

What acute treatments are available
    for headaches?   65

What happens when people take too many
    painkillers?   71

The principles of preventive treatment
    of headaches   79

What oral preventive treatments are available?   84

How does Botox help headaches?   96

What are CGRP monoclonal antibodies?   102

How is cluster headache treated?   107

What non-invasive neuromodulation options
    are available for headaches?   113

What lifestyle modifications can help
    reduce headaches?   119

What alternative treatments are known
    to help headaches?   133

Frequently Asked Questions

What can I expect out of a headache
    consultation?   139

Do I need a brain scan?   142

Are headaches hereditary?   147

Are headaches different in children?   150

Are people with headaches at risk of heart disease
   or stroke?   154

What role does the neck play in causing
   or exacerbating headaches?   158

What is the link between headaches and
   hormones?   162

How do you care for someone with headaches?   166

What does the future hold for those living
   with headaches?   169

What further resources are helpful for people
   with headaches, and their carers?   173

Acknowledgements   177
Endnotes   179
Index   181

Introduction

This book is the distillate of over twenty years' experience as a neurologist, both in the NHS and private practice in the UK. For most of that time, the primary focus of my practice has been headache. This book covers the headache basics (the common types of headache and how they are diagnosed), the science behind headaches, treatment options (from lifestyle modifications to surgery) and answers some of the most frequently asked questions about headaches.

This book is not just a self-help manual, though I hope that people who suffer from headaches, and those who care for them, will find it very useful in helping them understand headaches better, and in providing some practical steps to improve matters. It is written rather in the spirit of Oliver Sacks' book about migraine (now more than fifty years old) which aimed to explain what was known about the condition at the time, and to show people how multifaceted and extraordinary migraine could be. One of the values of Sacks' book was that it was the first popular account of the various components of migraine attacks in which people could read and recognise their experiences, and understand that what they were experiencing was in fact 'normal'. One of the most valuable aspects of talking to a clinician who looks after patients with migraine and other headache disorders, is that such a person can reassure patients that their experiences are not unique to them, that they are not imagining them, and that they do not presage or indicate the presence of any more dangerous neurological disorder. Migraine and other headache disorders can of course be serious enough in terms of the effect they have on people's quality of life; knowing that what you are experiencing is due to migraine or another headache disorder is an important step in improving that quality of life for many patients.

Finally, the advice contained in this book is intended to be applied to the management of headache disorders in general terms, and is not to be regarded as in any way a substitute for a proper consultation with a headache specialist, if appropriate. If after reading this book, you find that you do not need to have that consultation, then I have succeeded in what I set out to do, and if you do need to have that consultation, I hope you will be able to have a fuller, more constructive conversation, which will, over time, allow you to live better with your headaches.

The Basics

What is a headache?

'Begin at the beginning,' the King said gravely, 'and go on till you come to the end: then stop.'

Lewis Carroll (migraine sufferer),
Alice's Adventures in Wonderland (1865)[1]

To begin, therefore, at the beginning: what is a headache?

The International Association for the Study of Pain (IASP) defines pain as an 'unpleasant sensory and emotional experience associated with, or resembling that associated with, actual or potential tissue damage.' In the supporting notes, they state that pain is always a personal experience, influenced to varying degrees by biological, psychological and social factors. They further note that individuals learn the concept of pain through their life experiences, and stress that a person's report of an experience as pain should be respected. They also note that, while pain usually serves an adaptive role, it may have adverse effects on function, and social and psychological well-being.

In the simplest terms, therefore, a headache is a pain that affects the head or the face. Attempts to describe and define headache date back thousands of years, but ever since the 1980s the globally accepted method of classification is that devised by the International Headache Society (IHS), and embodied in its International Classification of Headache Disorders (ICHD), now in its third edition. This draws a fundamental distinction between primary headaches and secondary headaches.

Primary headaches are those caused by conditions that create the experience of pain from abnormal functioning of sensory processing systems within the brain. In primary headaches there is no 'actual or potential tissue damage' (though it often feels like there is); these headaches are unpleasant sensory and emotional experiences that may resemble those associated with tissue damage, though they often have features all of their own. The commonest primary headache is tension-type headache. The commonest debilitating primary headache, by far, is migraine. Much of this book will be concerned with migraine, its manifestations and its treatment. There are (at present count) another fourteen primary headache disorders, most of which are rare and under-diagnosed.

*

Secondary headaches arise from the stimulation of pain receptors in and around the head, face and neck; here there is 'actual or potential tissue damage'. The brain itself has no pain receptors, but the membranes that line the brain have them, as do cerebral blood vessels, muscles, joints, ligaments, tendons and other soft tissues. Secondary headaches are also common. Most of us get headaches if we have a cold or the flu.

It is generally the case that primary headaches will come and go in an intermittent, or episodic pattern, whereas secondary headaches will usually persist, at least until the underlying problem is dealt with, or resolves by itself. There are important exceptions to this general rule, but it is a useful starting point for diagnosis if you experience headaches, or are looking after someone who does. As we will see, there are a number of common misattributions, perhaps the most common of which is to misdiagnose migraine as either tension-type headache or 'sinus headache'.

The ICHD is the bible for headache specialists, but like the Bible it is long, full of lists, and prone to generate sects and controversies. The main purpose of creating the classification was to ensure uniformity in assessing patients for research trials, and it is important to remember that not everyone's headache has read the ICHD. People can have migraines without fulfilling the strict criteria listed in the document.

Migraine attacks can be longer or shorter than the typical duration; they can have other features not listed in the ICHD, or be largely bereft of those features.

Nonetheless, classification and diagnosis is important. Getting a diagnosis is the first step on the road to getting effective treatment, and learning how to live with headaches.

What type of headache do I have?

> *I keep six honest serving-men*
> *(They taught me all I knew);*
> *Their names are What and Why and When*
> *And How and Where and Who.*
>
> Rudyard Kipling, *Just So Stories*(1902)[2]

When diagnosing headaches, most of the relevant information lies in the history – that is, the description of the character and pattern of headaches. Most people can diagnose their own headaches correctly by paying attention to their own headache history.

Ask yourself a few simple questions:

What is the pattern of the headaches? Do they come and go? In other words, are they episodic headaches? Or are they there all the time, or pretty much so (chronic headaches)? If they come and go, how long do they typically last for? Minutes? Hours? Days?

How severe are your headaches? Are they mild enough that you can basically ignore them and get on with things? Or moderate – that is, bad enough to start to make it difficult for you to carry on with what you are doing, while remaining just about possible? Or severe – bad enough to stop you doing anything until the headache has passed?

Does anything happen when you get headaches? Do you feel sick? Do you find that lights or noises bother you, and make the pain worse? Does movement (such as shaking your head or running upstairs) make the headache worse? Do you experience any disturbances of your vision, or odd sensations in your head or body before or during the headache? Is there any redness or watering of the eye on the same side as the headache? Does your nose run or feel blocked?

If you have episodic headaches, then this relatively small amount of information will probably be enough to make a diagnosis, or at least a working diagnosis. There is a saying in medicine that 'common things are common'. The commonest forms of primary headache are tension-type headache and migraine. Essentially, if you experience recurrent mild, featureless headaches, then these are probably tension-type headaches, and if you suffer from recurrent moderate or severe headaches, with other features such as nausea or light sensitivity, then these are probably migraines. When I teach medical students or junior doctors about headaches, I tell them to start with this presumption; if they do, most of the time they will get the diagnosis right.

There are exceptions, of course, the most common of which is cluster headache, a condition that typically (though not invariably) will wake people at night with excruciatingly severe, one-sided pain in and around the eye, often associated with redness and watering of the eye on that side, and a restlessness that is very different from what people with migraine experience. We will talk more about cluster headache later on in this chapter (see page 12).

Chronic headaches can be a little more difficult to diagnose. They are often simply highly frequent or persistent forms of episodic disorders such as tension-type headache or migraine, but it is almost always the case that there are other things going on, either directly related to, or separate from, the underlying disorder, that become involved in driving the headache forward. Again, I will discuss what to look out for in people with chronic headaches in a later section (see page 18).

Rarely, persistent or chronic headaches are caused by other, potentially more severe underlying problems, and it is certainly sensible to seek medical opinion if you are getting headaches all the time, especially if they are associated with features such as fever, blurred or double vision, or limb weakness, or if you have a previous history of cancer, or have a weakened immune system. It's important to remember, however, that even if some of these features are present, it is still much more likely that your headache will be a benign, primary headache, than anything more worrisome.

Common primary headaches

> No one, of course, will dispute that kephalaia, as the phy-sicians call it, is a disease of the head. To say it briefly and in a concise sentence: this ailment is a chronic long-lasting and obstinate headache (kephalalgia), which flares up on minor provocation with such severe paroxysms that [the patients] cannot tolerate a noise, a loud voice or any bright light or motion but want to rest quietly in darkness because of the severity of the pain.
>
> Galen, *On the Affected Parts* (2nd century CE)[3]

Tension-type headache

Most people experience tension-type headaches at some point in their lives. This is a mild ache, not usually associated with any other features, that will go by itself, or with a simple painkiller such as paracetamol or ibuprofen. Most people can carry on their usual activities while they have a tension-type headache. They rarely cause any problems unless they become frequent or chronic.

Migraine

Migraine is by far the most common reason for people to experience recurrent, debilitating headaches. Later I devote a whole section to the question of what causes migraine, and why some people get them. Migraines typically cause moderate or severe head pain. They are often felt on one side of the head (the very name 'migraine' is a shortening of the Greek word 'hemicrania', meaning 'half-head'), but they can occur anywhere in the head, often sitting in the forehead or at the base of the back of the skull. They may have a throbbing or pulsating character. They are often preceded by, or associated with, pain in the neck, and more rarely elsewhere in the body.

Migraines are 'headaches plus', in that the pain is usually associated with one or more other features. These may include nausea, vomiting, sensitivity to lights, noises or smells. They are often made worse by any form of movement. Migraine headaches usually last hours, or even a few days. They can last a shorter time in children.

It is a common misconception (including amongst doctors) that you cannot be having a migraine if you do not have an aura.

This is a period of neurological dysfunction, usually affecting vision, that typically precedes the headache phase. But only about 25 to 30 per cent of people with migraine experience aura; far more people with migraine do not. The multifaceted manifestations of aura are the subjects of later sections.

About one in five people with migraine will get a warning that an attack is coming. This prodrome, or premonitory phase, may include symptoms such as fatigue, yawning, craving for sweet or salty foods, euphoria or frequent urination. At least as many people will experience a postdrome, or migraine hangover, during which, even though the pain has largely settled, they do not feel back to their usual selves, often struggling to concentrate or exert themselves physically.

In some cases aura, or even the prodrome and postdrome, can be more prolonged and debilitating than the headache itself. In other cases, the symptoms that occur in association with head pain – particularly nausea, light sensitivity or general malaise and 'brain fog' – can be more bothersome than the actual pain. Pain is the aspect of migraine that is most easily treated with medication; other symptoms can be more refractory to treatment.

Cluster headache

Cluster headache is a much rarer, but characteristic condition in which people experience invariably unilateral pain, in and around the eye, associated with activation of nerves over which we do not have voluntary control (autonomic nerves). This causes problems such as redness and watering of the eye on the side of the pain, running or blockage of the nose, swelling around the eye, drooping of the eyelid, excessive sweating and agitation or restlessness. People with cluster headache find it very difficult to stay still. They may rock to and fro, or pace around the house. In extreme cases they may actually hit their head against a wall to try to distract themselves from the pain. People with migraine may feel as if they want to do this, but they won't, because they know that any form of movement will make their pain worse, and they will generally lie as still as they can.

Dubbed the 'alarm clock headache', cluster headaches often wake people in the night. (They have gathered many spectacular names over the years, including ciliary neuralgia; erythromelalgia of the head; erythroprosopalgia of Bing; hemicrania angioparalytica; hemicrania neuralgiformis chronica; histaminic cephalalgia; Horton's headache; Harris-Horton's disease; migrainous neuralgia (of Harris); petrosal neuralgia (of Gardner); Sluder's neuralgia; sphenopalatine neuralgia; and vidian neuralgia.) Cluster attacks tend to be shorter than migraines, usually lasting no more than a couple of hours; but people can have multiple cluster attacks in one day.

Cluster headaches often come in bouts lasting a few weeks. There is a clear tendency for these bouts to come at certain times of year, often when day length changes in the spring or autumn. The diurnal and circannual rhythms of cluster headache may relate to activity in the hypothalamus – the bit of the brain that senses light and dark, and sets our body clock, and which is known to be involved in the systems that generate cluster attacks.

More men than women are affected by cluster headaches. It used to be thought that the ratio was as high as 9:1, but in recent years it has become clear that the condition has been under-diagnosed in women, so that ratio may be nearer 2–3:1. Migraine, by contrast, is much more common in women, at least 30 per cent of whom will experience it at some point in their lives.

Cluster headache is the most common of a class of primary headaches called the 'trigeminal autonomic cephalgias' that cause pain in the first division of the trigeminal nerve (the eye and forehead) and activation of the autonomic nerves. Paroxysmal hemicrania can be virtually identical to cluster headache, but the attacks are generally shorter (lasting minutes), and are responsive to a specific anti-inflammatory, indomethacin. SUNCT syndrome, and the related condition

SUNA, comprise brief but excruciating neuralgic pains in and around the eye, associated with prominent redness and watering of the eye (in the case of SUNCT), and other autonomic symptoms (in the case of SUNA). These conditions are very rare, similar to trigeminal neuralgia, and can be highly refractory to treatment.

Common secondary headaches

IV. Headache of nasal vasomotor reaction. V. Headache of delusional, conversion, or hypochondriacal states, VI. Nonmigrainous vascular headache, VII. Traction headache, VIII. Headache due to overt cranial inflammation. IX-XIII. Headache due to disease of ocular, aural, nasal, and sinus, dental or other cranial or neck structures.

Categories of secondary headache, according to the
1962 American Headache Society classification

Headaches caused by other medical conditions are not at all rare, and it is usually obvious when this is the case. Most people get a headache when they have an infection, for example. Headache is an almost invariable accompaniment to influenza, and even the common cold. In the last few years, there has been a lot of interest in headaches associated with coronavirus infection. Early studies that emerged from the epicentre of the pandemic in Wuhan indicated that about one in eight patients with Covid-19 experienced headache as a symptom. It is also clear, as we will discuss in the section on chronic headaches (see page 18), that infections can stir up or trigger a tendency to migraine or other primary headache disorders; this may account for the apparently high numbers of people developing persistent headaches after Covid-19, or after Covid vaccination.

Headaches can arise from any pain-sensitive structure in or around the head, face and neck. Many people believe that they are suffering from sinus headaches, but while acute inflammation of the sinuses can be excruciatingly painful, recurrent headaches that seem to be associated with sinus congestion are in fact unlikely to be related to sinus infection, but are more probably migraines (the feeling of congestion being due to the effect of a neurotransmitter released in migraine attacks that causes the blood vessels in the nasal passages to expand, thereby causing a localised tissue swelling that feels similar to that caused by a sinus infection). If you have a headache associated with a fever, nasal discharge and pain when you tap your forehead or cheek over the place where the pain is located, then the pain might indeed be coming from your sinuses; if not, it's probably not.

The neck, however, is a different matter. There is no doubt that people can experience head pain that arises from the neck. The soft tissues of the neck (the muscle, tendons and ligaments) and the vertebral facet joints all feed information into a bit of the brain (the trigeminocervical complex (TCC)) that is implicated in generating migraine pain, and which can almost certainly generate the experience of headache under other circumstances. An interesting study published in 2013 by a team in Los Angeles showed that, if they stimulated the high cervical nerve roots, this generated pain in the neck, but also pain higher in the head (and even at the front of the head, in an area served by a completely different set of nerves, though connected in the TCC in the brain). Frontal pain was much more likely to occur in people with a history of migraine, and it is likely to be the case that problems with the neck are one of the most common triggers that set off, or worsen, an intrinsic tendency to migraine. There is more on this in the FAQ section on the role of the neck in headache disorders (see page 158).

Headaches that arise directly from the neck can generally be recognised by the fact that certain movements bring on the pain, or that pressure on certain structures in the neck does so. Cervicogenic pain of this type can be transient (consisting of an electric shock-like or neuralgic quality), or more persistent, with a burning or itching character, arising from trapping of the occipital nerves as they pass through the muscle layers on their way down to the high cervical nerve roots. If those nerves fire off by themselves, this causes occipital neuralgia; if the signals are simply a little scrambled by pressure on the nerves at some point, the pain may have more of a neuropathic (or nerve-pain) quality. These cervicogenic headaches are usually associated with tenderness of some of the neck structures, and often with restriction of neck movements.

There are a multitude of other reasons why people may experience pain in the head. The modern-day successor to the 1962 classification mentioned at the start of this chapter (the third edition of the International Classification of Headache Disorders) lists dozens of pain syndromes originating in pain-sensitive structures in and around the head and neck, as well as from metabolic disturbances (such as excessively high or very low blood pressure, or abnormal levels of blood oxygen or other constituents), the presence of withdrawal of drugs (prescribed or otherwise) and so on. In most cases these causes will emerge in the course of usual history-taking and examination, but in some cases they will only be found if the right investigations are requested and relevant results obtained. Diagnosing primary headaches (even rare varieties) can usually be done on the history alone; unusual secondary headaches may be harder work.

What causes chronic headaches?

> But although this Distemper most grievously afflicting this
> noble Lady, above twenty years (when I saw her) having
> pitched its tents near the confines of the Brain, had so long
> besieged its regal tower, yet it had not taken it: for the sick
> Lady, being free from a Vertigo, swimming in the Head,
> Convulsive Distempers, and any Soporiferous symptom,
> found the chief faculties of her soul sound enough.
>
> Thomas Willis, writing about Lady Anne Conway,
> *Two Discourses of the Soul of Brutes Which*
> *Is The Vital and Sensitive Soul of Man* (1672)[4]

When trying to work out what is causing chronic headaches, it is important to start at the beginning.

The pattern of how chronic headaches start can be crucial in sorting out what is causing them. Did you have episodic headaches before you started to get more frequent or chronic headaches? Did things build up steadily from a point where you were getting occasional headaches to a point where you were getting them all the time? Or did they start suddenly one day, and just never go away? If they started suddenly, then what were the circumstances in which that happened? Was there any particular event – a head injury, an infection, or anything else that might give a clue? What has been the pattern since then? Have things got steadily worse, or has it reached a plateau and just not improved? Are there periods of remission or improvement?

It is then useful to think about the character of the headaches. Are they the same day after day, or are there bad days, and less bad days? If there is a baseline low-level headache, what is that like? Does the pain change during the day? Is it there when you wake up in the morning, or does it come on as the day goes on? What are the headaches like at their worst? Are there any features, for example, of migraine, or any other primary headache disorder?

Out of all of this, there are two common patterns that emerge. The first is a pattern epitomised by (and most commonly due to) a condition that was christened 'transformed migraine' in the 1980s by the American headache expert Ninan T. Mathew. This term has rather fallen out of favour in recent years, but it captures the evolution from an episodic to a chronic form of migraine that is quite a common process. This evolution can happen for a number of reasons. Sometimes it is just migraine doing what migraine does, but in other cases it may be driven by factors such as the overuse of painkillers, the secondary effects of migraine on neck pain and sleep (which can set up a vicious cycle that winds up migraine attacks), or other external factors. Over the years, for example, obesity, depression, anxiety and other medical problems have been shown to be associated, at least, with this type of progressive headache. This kind of transformation can happen with other primary headache disorders, but it is much rarer than with migraine.

The other common pattern is what has been dubbed in the headache world, 'new daily persistent headache'. This is not a diagnosis as such, but a descriptive term for a headache syndrome characterised by the development of a headache one day that then never goes away. It is an important pattern to recognise, because within this category lie most of the more serious reasons for people to get headaches. Theoretically one cannot diagnose this syndrome until people have had 'a headache' for more than three months. There are people who get occasional runs of migraines that may go on for a week or two, and of course bouts of cluster headache will typically last for a few weeks, or a small number of months. If the headaches have persisted beyond this timescale, or even if they haven't but are getting steadily worse, then they do warrant assessment. Having said that, it remains the case that the vast majority of people with this type of headache do not have a serious underlying neurological problem, other than a chronic headache disorder.

One of the most common scenarios is that a person who has previously had episodic migraine, or even just a family history of the condition, suddenly starts to experience regular headaches after a minor head injury, an infection, or even a vaccination. Why this happens to some people, and not others, is not known. This phenomenon has been seen widely in recent years with large numbers of people contracting Covid, and/or having Covid vaccinations, but it is not at all specific to the coronavirus. Whilst this reaction to an often innocuous trigger is uncommon, when large numbers of people were being exposed to such triggers at the same time, a small tidal wave of people with persistent headaches ensued. This was all made much worse in April 2021 by the nocebo effect (that is, the opposite of the placebo effect, whereby the expectation of a negative outcome creates that outcome) engendered by reports of life-threatening blood clots following administration of the AstraZeneca Covid vaccine, leading to Accident and Emergency departments being temporarily overrun by people with headaches. Fortunately simple measures were rapidly devised to sort the worried well from those with serious pathology, and the panic died down. The natural history of persistent migraines set off in this way, is generally that they will persist for weeks or even months, before gradually starting to improve, eventually settling back to the patient's previous baseline. In a small number of cases, however, things never seem to improve; it was these patients, who could pinpoint the day that their headache had started, and were still suffering years later, who were first given the diagnosis 'new daily persistent headache'; for this reason, this condition was for many years considered the most refractory of all headache types to treatment, but over time it has become apparent that, like most headache disorders, there is a spectrum of severity, at one end of which people can suffer unremitting headaches for years or even decades.

These types of headache are very rarely life threatening, but they can have an enormous adverse effect on people's quality of life. It is important to try to understand what causes them, and perhaps more importantly what perpetuates them, in individual cases, so that the best possible treatment can be found.

When does having headaches become an illness?

> *To have pain is to have* certainty; *to hear about pain is to have* doubt.
>
> Elaine Scarry, *The Body in Pain* (1985)[5]

Pretty much everybody gets headaches from time to time. Most of those headaches are mild, featureless, tension-type headaches, but in some cases the headaches will be more severe, and bring other symptoms along with them. When do headaches turn from being minor inconveniences to something more problematic? When, in other words taken from the lexicon of medicine, do they turn from being normal, to pathological?

Historians and philosophers of medicine have debated the essential nature of illness and disease, how this has been constructed and understood through the ages. In most ancient societies, including Chinese, Indian and Greco-Roman, disease was understood as resulting from a lack of balance, both within the body itself, and between the body and the world around it. This conception of disease persists in the understanding of illnesses such as diabetes, where the fundamental problem is an excess of a normal substance – sugar – in the body. The main challenge to this way of understanding disease came in the nineteenth century with the advent of the germ theory, which held that disease was due to the influence of microscopic organisms – bacteria, viruses and so on – on the body. In this conception, disease is something alien, other, an invader that needs to be expelled from the body, or prevented from entering in the first place. Drawing distinctions between normal and pathological seems straightforward in the latter case, until one starts to think about the concept of 'good' bacteria (probiotic bacteria) that normally live within our gut, in harmony and health.

As the philosopher Hari Cavel points out in her book on the phenomenology of illness, even a mild headache can 'bring to light the tacit sense in which all projects ultimately rest on bodily abilities'. But she points out that there is a fundamental difference between a mild headache and more serious illness: 'Minor ailments fit within, and hence do not disrupt, one's being in the world. Serious illness modifies the ill person's way of being.' A tension-type headache might be a temporary frustration, but it does not permanently and radically modify people's bodily experiences and self-understanding in the way that more serious illness can:

> even simple bodily disruptions, like a headache, may still reveal to us the contingency of our bodily being, although they do not modify the structure of experience in the way that deep disruption does. The headache may not be severe and it is transient. But even a simple headache disrupts the activity one is immersed in and thus reveals how our immersion in the everyday world is dependent on bodily integrity.

What, then, characterises more serious illness?

Cavel discusses the work of the philosopher Kay Toombs, who herself suffered from a chronic neurological illness (multiple sclerosis). Toombs strived to define the essential features of illness. She defined these in terms of five losses: the loss of wholeness, the loss of certainty, the loss of control, the loss of the freedom to act and the loss of a familiar world. Applying these to headache disorders, the idea of the loss of wholeness comprises a whole raft of problems around bodily impairment, resulting in headache sufferers no longer being able to take their bodies for granted or ignore them; headaches thwart plans, impede choices and render certain actions impossible.

For patients with headache disorders, the loss of certainty is common; headaches often cause capricious, unpredictable interruptions to life, and even at a low frequency, this may engender anxiety and apprehension. The familiar world – in which one can reliably carry on normal activities, work and play – is disrupted. Future plans have to be adjusted or abandoned. People with severe or refractory headache disorders often feel that they have lost control; their place in the world seems increasingly unpredictable, and they may ultimately find that they have lost the freedom to act as they wish (even in discussions with doctors and other healthcare professionals).

Ultimately, as Cavel points out, illness is:

> the loss of opportunities, possibilities, and openness. It is the closure of a previously open future: future possibilities close down as illness progresses. But it is also the closure of the present: current daily activities lose their habitual aspect and become carefully planned and demanding. What could once be done unthinkingly, with no planning and marginal effort, is now an explicit task, requiring thought, attention, and a pronounced effort.

This leads to 'an ongoing lamentation for things lost, gone, given up on. Life becomes a set of constraints, a levy charged at every twist and turn, making day trips expensive, outings exhausting, travelling not feasible, spontaneity overridden by physical constraints.' Patients suffering from chronic headache disorders may eventually find themselves in what Cavel terms 'the world of "no longer able to", the world of inability to be, or do, so many things.'

The invisibility and incommunicability of the experience of headache brings additional problems. Cavel writes about breathlessness, noting that the 'distress and sense of impending suffocation, the panic bubbling up in severe breathlessness, the sense of loss of control, are entirely internal, impenetrable, . . . invisible . . . An observer can see the person standing still and panting, the laboured breathing – but these do not really convey the subjective sensation of severe distress.' The same can be said for patients suffering from migraine or cluster headache. Cavel notes that the 'ability of a healthy person to understand the constricted experiential space of the breathless person is limited because of the lack of a shared experiential background.' For headache sufferers the situation may be worse, because most people have experienced headaches, and may therefore consciously or subconsciously assume that they understand and share their experience of headache, when in reality they may not.

The historian of pain Elaine Scarry's statement on the role of doubt in pain, presented at the head of this chapter, will resonate with many headache patients, who can find that they suffer from a double dose of doubt: doubt that they experience pain at all, and doubt that the effects they ascribe to their pain are real and commensurate with the level of pain that they report.

Doubt brings in its wake stigma. Sufferers' experiences of migraine stigma have recently been shown to be strongly associated with their migraine outcomes, and the presence of other psychiatric symptoms. They are independently associated with migraine disability and emotion-related quality of life in migraine sufferers. Migraine stigma is an important contributor to the relationship between headache frequency and migraine outcomes, and it is incumbent on all those who treat patients with migraine and other headache disorders to recognise this, and do their best to counter stigma.

The science bit

Where does the pain of headache come from?

> I wanted to describe chronic migraines as proof
> that the chemical operations
> in my large brain
> are working in an orderly fashion.
> I wanted to begin:
> My hands are not enough to hold my head.
>
> From 'I Describe a Migraine', Iman Mersel (2006)[6]

When thinking about the WHO definition of pain as an experience that derives from actual or potential tissue damage, it becomes relatively easy to see where the pain of most secondary headaches comes from. If your headache comes from a problem with your sinuses, or your jaw, or with your neck, it is straightforward to understand how pain signals arising from sensory receptors in those areas may end up causing you the experience of pain that, for the most part, localises to the place from where the pain arises. Pain receptors do not generally like to be traumatised, either by direct physical pressure, by localised inflammation (such as happens in sinus infections), or by repeated over-strain of muscles, ligaments, or other soft tissues (such as happens in the neck). At a brain level, sensory signals from the trigeminal nerve (which serves pretty much everything from the crown of the head forward as far down as the angle of the jaw and the chin) and the top three cervical nerve roots in the neck (which serve the back of the head, the neck and the shoulders, respectively) are processed in an area called the trigeminocervical complex (TCC). This is a complex sensory processing area, which is constantly receiving information from the whole of the head and the neck, and also sending out signals in return. Most of that activity does not reach our global workspace of consciousness – in other words, we are simply not aware of it – but pain can break through the systems that normally keep this complex from sending signals up into higher centres within the brain, and when that happens, we feel pain.

The nature of sensory processing within the TCC means that abnormal inputs from one part of the head and neck can cause the experience of pain elsewhere. Pain arising from the neck can be felt in the forehead, and vice versa. This type of referred pain is not significantly different from that caused by the convergence of sensory signals at the level of the spinal cord, which can result in pain from the diaphragm being felt at the tip of the shoulder, or from an inflamed appendix being felt (initially at least) rather vaguely throughout the whole of the abdomen.

So far, so straightforward. But what about primary headache disorders, such as tension-type headache, migraine or cluster headache? In these conditions, there is no input into the TCC, only an output. In patients with primary headaches, abnormal sensory signals from the head and neck may exacerbate those headache disorders, but they are not the cause of the pain. As mentioned above, the TCC sends out signals as well as receiving them. The most relevant output for primary headache disorders is activity in nerves that supply the extracranial blood vessels that line the surface of the brain or the interior of the skull (such as the meningeal arteries or dural veins). It was demonstrated in the 1930s and 1940s that electrical stimulation of these blood vessels (in volunteers who were woken during brain surgery for the experiment) caused an experience of pain indistinguishable from migraine or other primary headaches. Functional imaging techniques such as positron emission tomography (PET) and functional magnetic resonance imaging (MRI) scanning showed in the 1990s and 2000s that the first thing to happen in a migraine or cluster headache was activation of the area in the brainstem that contains the TCC. This increases activity in the nerves that take information to the extracranial blood vessels, which then increases the release of vasoactive neurotransmitters into those vessels. These in turn stimulate trigeminal sensory nerves, which take information back in a loop, via the trigeminal ganglion, to the TCC. This loop is always active at a low level, but in primary headaches it starts to run hot. Eventually this generates additional signals within the TCC that over-ride the upstream control mechanisms (located in the midbrain and hypothalamus) that normally prevent us from being aware of all this sensory activity. It is likely that the fundamental (genetic) reason why some people are headachy, and others not so, revolves around the effectiveness, or otherwise, of these descending control mechanisms. The TCC starts to send signals up to the thalamus, and ultimately to the sensory cortex, at which point we become conscious of the process – we have a headache.

Studies of brain connectivity (that is, of the activity of circuits that connect different regions of the brain together) over the last decade indicate that, in between migraine attacks, most brain networks are more active in people with migraine than in those who do not have the condition. This accords with older studies that used electrophysiological techniques, which showed that 'migraine brains' do not habituate to abnormal sensory inputs in the same way that other people's brains do. This all changes during an attack, before resetting in the postdrome. These changes in connectivity and habituation follow a cyclical pattern, building to a peak just before a migraine comes. In some people this can manifest as an almost rhythmical pattern of attacks. More often it simply provides a background against which triggers will sometimes set off attacks, whilst at other times they will not. This intrinsic rhythmicity of headache processes in the brain explains why lifestyle and trigger management may not always succeed in keeping headaches completely under control.

Additional inputs into that system may explain some of the features of migraine and cluster headache. In the case of the former, for example, many people experience photophobia: that is, a worsening of their headache pain by exposure to normal levels of light. It has been shown, in elegant work performed by a team under the American neurologist Rami Burstein, that there are direct connections between the retina and the thalamus. These connections normally serve a protective function, alerting the brain to the possibility that very bright light may damage the eye. In migraine, however, normal signals passing along this connection are believed to ramp up the signals passing through the thalamus on their way to the sensory cortex. In cluster headache, there is excessive activity of the sphenopalatine ganglion (the SPG, which is one of the relay stations in the loop between the TCC and the extracranial blood vessels), which in turn triggers the autonomic nerves over which we have no voluntary control. This leads to characteristic features of cluster and related trigeminal autonomic cephalgias, including redness and watering of the eye, drooping of the eyelid, excess sweating and agitation. This is the same system that is activated by chillies or other spicy foods, causing the characteristic 'chilli sniffle'; in those cases, symptoms are caused by capsaicin in the chilli stimulating specific receptors in the SPG; in cluster headache it is the intrinsic release of vasoactive neurotransmitters that is responsible.

The experience of pain when there is no actual tissue damage in primary headache disorders begs the question of why these systems should be so prone to work in this way. What is the possible evolutionary benefit to humankind of experiencing so much head pain without a clear and obvious reason behind it? There is no good answer to this question, but it is possibly instructive to note that many of the circumstances in which migraines, for example, are triggered (missing a meal, poor sleep, menstruation) are those in which the resilience and reserves of the body may be compromised. The behaviour associated with having a migraine attack – retreating into a dark, quiet place, and sleeping – may act to restore the body's metabolic equanimity. Migraine and other headaches may be a response to periods of extreme stress (in the broadest sense). In this regard, it is fascinating to realise that the process that causes migraine aura – cortical spreading depression (more of which in the chapter "What causes aura?" see page 41) – is highly conserved through evolution, and acts in insects such as locusts to turn off the brain in reaction to heat stress, preserving life by engendering a hibernation-like state.

It is easy to understand why so many people with migraine and other headache disorders assume that their headaches must arise from serious problems within the brain and body as a whole. Our early experiences of pain – falling over and scraping our knee as a child, for example – are generally characterised by an obvious sequence of cause and effect. When we get headaches, we cannot see the cause, but that does not mean that we do not believe that there is one to be found. This is one of the reasons why people may – paradoxically – become disappointed when presented with brain scans and other tests that are normal. It is also why explaining about the nature of primary headache disorders is so important, so that people do not embark upon long, expensive and fruitless tests for abnormalities that can never be found. Primary headaches are, for the most part, a software problem, not a hardware problem. Accepting and understanding that is an important part of learning how to live with headaches.

What is CGRP, and what does it have to do with headache?

CGRP may be of considerable importance in the regulation of cerebral blood flow and in the migraine syndrome.
Lars Edvinsson, *Trends in Neurosciences* (1985)[7]

In the last few years, a number of new treatments for migraine and other headaches have started to emerge, all of which in some way affect the function of a neurotransmitter called CGRP (calcitonin gene-related peptide). What does CGRP do, and why does influencing this help manage headaches?

CGRP is a protein that acts as a neurotransmitter, both within the brain itself and elsewhere within the body. It holds the distinction of being the first protein the existence of which was predicted from its genetic code, before it was actually found *in vivo*. In the early 1980s, researchers working on calcitonin, a protein involved in the actions of the thyroid gland, isolated the gene responsible for encoding it, but noticed that the gene seemed to contain too much information simply for this purpose, and they hypothesised that the gene might also contain the code for another protein, hence calcitonin gene-*related* peptide (a peptide being a portion of a protein molecule). CGRP was subsequently discovered to be widely distributed within the brain and body, and was fairly rapidly found to have potent effects in dilating blood vessels. Work done by, amongst others, the scientist Lars Edvinsson, studying the cerebral circulation as part of a research group based in Edinburgh in the 1980s, suggested that it might be important in protecting the body against the effects of blood vessel constriction. As it was already known at the time that the calibre of blood vessels changed during migraine attacks, Edvinsson speculated early on that CGRP might be important for migraine.

At a meeting in Sweden in 1987, Edvinsson met a young Australian clinician-scientist called Peter Goadsby. Edvinsson and Goadsby found that they had interests in common, particularly in the question of how blood flow in migraine was controlled by neural mechanisms in the brain. Working together over the next few years, they demonstrated that CGRP levels were elevated in people having migraine and cluster headache attacks, and that as the attacks were treated, CGRP levels fell. They further demonstrated how the then-novel drug sumatriptan worked by blocking the release of CGRP, which was something of a surprise as it had been assumed that the therapeutic effect of sumatriptan was mediated through a different neurotransmitter – serotonin.

Further evidence supporting the importance of CGRP accrued over the next few years. A team led by the prominent Danish headache expert Jes Olesen (who had initially been sceptical about the role of CGRP) showed that giving migraine sufferers infusions of CGRP triggered migraine attacks in a high proportion of cases. Much of migraine science between the mid 1990s and mid 2010s was focused on understanding where CGRP is located in the brain systems involved in migraine physiology, how it is released in migraine attacks, and what the effect of blocking that might be. Pharmaceutical companies quickly picked up on the importance of CGRP, and started to develop new drugs that might impact upon its release. In the early 2000s, a series of drugs were developed that antagonised the effect of CGRP more directly than the triptans. Several of these went through the clinical trial process, and one of them (telcagepant) was set to be licensed and released for widespread use in early 2008. At the last minute, however, the drug was withdrawn because a small number of patients who had been given the drug in the clinical trials were found to have developed significant abnormalities of their liver function. From a point where it looked like the future of migraine might be 'gepants' (the suffix attached to all of this class of CGRP antagonists), it suddenly became (as Goadsby joked at an international headache congress, though only his idiomatic English-speaking audience got the joke) 'pants'. As we will see in a subsequent section, the gepants have made a comeback in the early 2020s.

The story of CGRP and migraine did not die with telcagepant, however. Useful drugs do not always start out as such. One transformation, seen time and time again in the modern history of medicine, is the evolution from laboratory tool to pharmaceutical phenomenon. Classic examples include penicillin, which was initially used by Alexander Fleming to get rid of fast-growing bacteria so he could study the more fastidious types in which he was interested; and physostigmine, the first effective treatment for myasthenia gravis, developed by the physiologist Otto Loewi to make it easier to detect the neurotransmitter acetylcholine. It was the remarkable female physician Mary Walker who first applied it in 1934 to the treatment of patients with what had previously been an incurable neurological disorder.

In the early 2000s, as part of the research toolkit devised to try to understand where CGRP could be found in the brain and body, researchers created artificial specific ('monoclonal') antibodies (see also 'What are CGRP monoclonal antibodies?' in the Treatments chapter on page 65) that precisely and exclusively attached themselves to the CGRP molecule or its receptor. The first report of a monoclonal antibody (mAb) specific to CGRP appears in the scientific literature in 2007, where it was described as a CGRP 'scavenger', used to investigate the distribution and function of the molecule in the brain and peripheral nervous system. This first mAb was made by a company called Rinat Neuroscience, based in Palo Alto, California. It was subsequently acquired by Pfizer, and licensed on to TEVA Pharmaceuticals.

The penny dropped quickly. By 2013 the journal *Nature Reviews Drug Discovery* was trumpeting the 'comeback' of the 'flagging migraine target' CGRP, as mAbs advanced into Phase II clinical trials. Within a year the headline was 'Anti-CGRP antibodies for migraine turn industry heads', as the first Phase II studies appeared in the journal *The Lancet Neurology*. By 2015, it was 'CGRP antibodies: the Holy Grail for migraine prevention?'

After the publication of Phase III trials of three mAbs (erenumab, fremanezumab and galcanezumab) in 2018, applications were quickly made to the FDA in the United States and to the EMA in Europe for the mAbs to be licensed. A fourth mAb (eptizenumab) was approved by the FDA in 2020. Marketing authorisation was granted in Europe (at that time still including the UK) for erenumab (Aimovig) in 2018, galcanezumab (Emgality) in November 2018, fremanezumab (Ajovy) in 2019, and eptizenumab (Vyepti) in 2022. The names of mAbs may seem a mouthful, but they follow established rules of nomenclature. The -umab ending of erenumab indicates that it is a human antibody, whereas the -zumab endings of the other antibodies indicate that they are humanised. The original Rinat Neuroscience mAb, for example, was created in rabbits, parts of the variable regions being modified to prevent the antibodies being rejected by the human immune system. In practice, this makes little difference, as does the fact that erenumab binds to the CGRP receptor, while the other mAbs bind to the molecule itself. The results of the Phase III studies are pretty consistent across the board: the mAbs have the potential to reduce the frequency and severity of migraines in anyone who is having more than four migraine days each month.

What is aura?

Ambushed by
pins and needles
of light . . .
by jagged
voices . . . strobes . . .
the sanctuary is taken
from within.
I am betrayed by
the fractured
senses.

From 'Migraine', Linda Pasten (1994)[8]

It was a hot summer's day. The year was 1981. I was playing cricket in my parents' back garden, when the ball ran away down a gentle slope, coming to rest under a small clump of shrubs. I squeezed under the bushes and scrabbled among the crisp fallen leaves for the ball. After a couple of minutes of searching, I emerged, ball in hand, back into the sunlight. As my eyes re-accustomed themselves to the light, I noticed something amiss. There, near the centre of my vision, was a small glowing dot. Wherever I looked, there was the dot, flickering and pulsing, unmistakably organic, mysterious. I started to feel slightly light-headed and queasy. The dot, I realised, was growing, slowly but steadily. The edges were taking on a sharp, jagged appearance, expanding outwards to the side and downwards in a ragged crescent. The sharpness had a scintillating quality to it, bright and silver, yet somehow containing colours, flickering in and out of my vision a thousand times each second. As the dot grew into a crescent, the world inside it simply disappeared. I looked at the house, and then at the line of tall pines that grew next to it. Whatever I looked at disappeared, and was surrounded on two, almost three sides by a flashing boundary.

I headed inside to find my parents. As I did so I became aware that the centre of my vision was clearing. The blind spot was following the pulsing crescent out into the peripheries of my vision. That was reassuring, but I found that as the crescent expanded outwards it began to creep upwards to fill the whole of the right half of my vision. I began to feel slightly disorientated, as if I was becoming detached from the world around me. I found my mother in the kitchen. 'I can't see properly,' I began. 'I've got this flashing light in my eye. It's getting bigger and bigger.' My mother looked up from her cookbooks. 'That's just a migraine,' she said. 'Don't worry, it'll soon pass.' And pass it did. The crescent kept on expanding until it disappeared, and my vision recovered. As it did so there was a brief moment in which everything felt brighter and clearer than normal, but that feeling passed almost as soon as I noticed it. Afterwards I vaguely recall having a headache.

I had just had my first experience of a migraine aura, something to which it transpired both my parents were prone. The first detailed description of aura was written by Dr Hubert Airy, presented to the Royal Society in London in 1870, and published shortly afterwards in the *Philosophical Transactions* of that Society. Airy collated previous accounts of the condition, including several published in the nineteenth century by eminent men of science: William Hyde Wollaston, Sir David Brewster and Airy's father, George, the Astronomer Royal. While the scientists were predominantly interested in the visual phenomena as potentially instructive in the broader context of the increasing interest in the physical basis of light, the laws of optics and the psychology of visual perception, Hubert Airy approached the phenomena from a more purely medical point of view, commencing his account by asking, perhaps only semi-rhetorically, why members of his profession had not taken more interest in such a common and fascinating phenomenon.

Airy's first migraine occurred in 1854. He wrote in his diary that it was 'like a fortified town with bastions all round it, these bastions being coloured most gorgeously'. He coined the neologism 'teichopsia' (Greek for 'town-wall vision') to describe the phenomenon. Airy also compared the phenomena to a 'cloud', or a 'thick liquid all alive': 'boiling', 'seething', full of 'turbulence and trembling'. He also used a military metaphor – an increasingly common trope in medicine from the 1860s onwards, and which still pervades migraine literature (both lay and technical) to the present day – referring to 'attacks' extending and spreading outwards to 'invade the more distant parts of the field of vision'. Occasionally he observes 'the rudiments of a fresh attack, beginning nearly where the first began, and sometimes advancing so far as to exhibit its bastioned margin'. With this sense of being under attack comes an oppression, a horror of the experience: 'I have seen a person,' Airy wrote, 'terribly subject to these attacks, shudder at the very name, and turn away from a drawing of the ugly sight, quite content to bear serious illness "if only the 'half-blindness' would keep away."'

My aura experience seems to have been very similar to Airy's, if the illustrations that accompany his paper are anything to go by, but ours was not the sole pattern of visual aura. Wollaston, for example, had described a 'shaded darkness without definite outline' which moved from the centre of his vision upwards towards the left. Brewster experienced a blindness or 'insensibility to distinct impressions' to one side or other of the centre of his vision, extending irregularly outwards on the same side. Wollaston and Brewster's descriptions epitomise the contrasting features of aura: 'positive' symptoms – that is, the presence of something in the vision, such as Wollaston's 'darkness' – and 'negative' symptoms – the absence of something, exemplified by Brewster's 'insensibility'. Positive visual symptoms are those things we see that are not actually there:

spectral hallucinations, moving, growing, changing and then fading away; negative visual symptoms are blind spots, holes or fractures in the visual world. By strict definition, aura should comprise both positive and negative symptoms, but not all aura follows the rules.

In addition, while aura is commonly visual, other symptoms can occur, such as disturbances of speech or memory. As early as 1870, in his monumental monograph on migraine, the physician Edward Liveing expanded the concept to include disturbances of sensation, balance and vertigo. A century later, the neurologist Oliver Sacks characterised aura symptoms under the headings of specific visual, tactile and other sensory hallucinations; general alterations of sensory threshold and excitability; alterations in level of consciousness and muscular tone; alterations of mood and affect; and disorders of higher functions (such as perception, memory or speech). Examples of the more unusual types of aura experience are given below (see page 46).

Typically, aura precedes the headache phase of migraine, but in some cases aura develops during the headache, or as it settles, or comes on its own, without any pain or other symptoms. There is no scan or blood test to diagnose aura. Everything is in the history – the description of the experience that the patient provides – while the doctor encourages, questions, clarifies and interprets. It can be difficult for people to find words to describe their experiences: not everyone has the benefit of Airy's gift for description, or his classical education. One patient, for example, was referred to me with 'blackouts', but when I delved into her symptoms, I found that she was experiencing blurring and stars in her vision, lasting ten minutes at a time, followed by a sick headache, and was not losing consciousness at all.

What are the varieties of visual aura?

> . . . *every six weeks or so, a school of small silver fish swim from the periphery across my retina . . . The fish in my head skitter and swarm, all together now, like neon tetras: magnetized, of one mind . . . And when the lights appear, flashing and blue against the purple sky lining my forehead, I brace myself. These are lights of distress.*
>
> Holly Harden, *On Migraines* (2002)[9]

Many of my patients describe scintillating zigzag crescents that are identical in many respects to those experienced and drawn by Hubert Airy. I often show people Airy's pictures online, and on several occasions, this has elicited an audible gasp of recognition from those previously unaware of the nature of their experience. Where one cannot simply point at a drawing and say, 'Yes, that is what I see,' it becomes necessary to translate a visual, tactile or visceral experience into words; and for this, simile and analogy are indispensable. One sporting patient described the phenomenon as being a zigzag visual disturbance 'like half a rugby ball', fluctuating in size. Another experienced distortion of his central vision 'like a crunched-up piece of silver paper'. Not infrequently patients will describe aura as like looking through a kaleidoscope (this pleases me when I recall that it was Sir David Brewster who invented this device) or a 'broken mirror'. One memorably told me her auras were 'like barbed wire with a blank in the middle'. Another described a shimmering circle 'like a mirage' in the distance, which grew to fill much of the left side of her vision over about ten minutes. In another case I recorded a 'fine lightning bolt in the inferior left visual field, which may oscillate in and out of vision'. This grew steadily to a 'moving, jelly-like, fractal glimmering', which became 'like a see-through water ripple'. Another patient gave a very similar description, comparing the symptoms to the 'sun setting glistening on rippling water'. The similarity of aura to patterns in water can sometimes be inverted, as in the case of the patient who described her aura as what one might obtain by 'pouring a black fluid into water'. Less frequently the scintillations are horizontal or vertical, drifting across or out of the visual fields. Typically, small disturbances grow to fill the whole of the vision, but not infrequently the disturbances begin at the peripheries of vision and move inwards, occasionally filling the whole of the visual fields as they do so.

The visual phenomena of aura can be simpler still: patients describe black patches, a loss of focus, a 'blotchy hand blocking vision', blurred vision, silver lines, a whitening of vision or a haze or fuzziness. One patient with peripheral cloudiness of vision described it as being 'blinkered'. Others speak of developing a form of tunnel vision. Sometimes vision sparkles, often at the peripheral edge of awareness, almost out of the visual world, everything becoming glittering and bright. Sometimes the effect is that of fireworks or windmills in or just at the edge of vision. Other patients describe more complex visual changes such as swirling colourful formations or circular flashing rainbows. One patient described small spots in her vision, coloured 'light yellow and cream or dark blue to black', like after-images of bright lights; occasionally she would have rather larger splodges of colour which could last for up to ten minutes before fading away. Another described 'yellow and red flashing spots or lights'; yet another described how the left side of her visual fields would become 'like a turbine spinning round in a circle', appearances which she called 'holographic'. Not every attack necessarily manifests itself in exactly the same way, as in the patient who experienced a whole range of visual distortions, from a simple inability to focus, to more complicated patterns such as zigzags, concentric circles or geometric shapes, often in luminous, bright colours.

Occasionally there is no positive component at all, patients suddenly realising that a portion of their visual world is missing. This loss of function also occurs in strokes and transient ischaemic attacks, but curiously, in such conditions patients are often completely unaware of their visual deficit until they start to bump into things on the side they cannot see. In migraine, the affected area is usually smaller and typically evolves over a few minutes, and it is perhaps this that allows people to appreciate the missing portion of their vision.

Other disturbances of vision can be yet more complex. Patients can complain of letters dancing, jumping or swirling on the page, fading of the colour and acuity of vision in one part of their visual world, loss of depth perception (the world seeming somehow flat during their aura) or visual persistence (also called palinopsia): that is, a sense that 'someone presses the pause button' on vision and turns the sound off; in such cases, when patients close their eyes and open them again, everything may be back to normal or have started to move, but only in slow motion. In some cases it is the *processing* of visual information that is affected, such as the ability to extract meanings from shapes: about one such patient I wrote, 'He describes how he can trace a shape or letters onto a piece of paper and then suddenly realise that they form a word. He may also look at his pen in his hand and be unable to think what it is or what it is used for.'

Very rarely visual aura can become frightening. In one case, a fairly typical history of visual aura ('visual flickering associated with cracked vision') developed into a feeling that the 'bed is going up and down or the walls are going in and out'; this same patient had episodes where she became 'convinced that there are people in the house or her sister was talking in her ear' or 'experienced a feeling that someone was there next to her which made her feel scared . . . associated with a feeling of being paralysed, as though she could not shout out'. On another particularly disconcerting occasion she 'had an episode where she felt as she had gone downstairs and opened the door to see mudflats outside, when she had not in fact moved from her bed at all.' Such florid and complex hallucinations are rare in migraine, and will, not surprisingly, raise concerns in both patients and those who look after them about an underlying psychosis or other mental health disorder, but the history of such episodes occurring solely in the context of a developing migraine attack will usually allow the correct diagnosis to be made.

What other types of aura are there?

> *'Curiouser and curiouser!' cried Alice . . . 'now I'm opening out like the largest telescope that ever was! Good-bye feet!'*
> Lewis Carroll, *Alice's Adventures in Wonderland* (1865)[10]

Most people who get migraine with aura experience visual symptoms. After this, the second commonest form of aura is a disturbance of sensation. Like visual aura, sensory aura typically consists of a combination of positive and negative symptoms, in this case parasthesiae (tingling, pins and needles) and numbness (loss of sensation). Again, like visual aura, these symptoms will typically evolve over a matter of minutes, often starting in the fingers of one hand, spreading up the arm and into the face on that side, or vice versa. The whole of one side of the body can be affected, or in other cases just isolated patches. The most commonly affected areas are those which are most extensively represented in the sensory regions of the brain – the hands, lips, tongue and face. Involvement of the torso, the legs and specific areas, such as the tip of the nose, is less typical, but not unheard of. In some cases the symptoms can be very restricted – for example, one of my patients experiences tingling in the fifth finger that only ever spreads as far as the third finger of the same hand. In such cases it can sometimes be difficult to distinguish sensory aura from the consequences of the trapping or dysfunction of a peripheral nerve or spinal nerve root. In the above case, the history of repeated episodes of disturbance followed by a migrainous headache eventually made it clear what was going on.

Sensory aura often follows visual aura, as the process that causes aura spreads forward from the visual cortex into other areas of the brain, but sensory disturbances can be isolated, or associated with other non-visual manifestations of aura. When there is visual aura beforehand and headache afterwards, it is easy to make the diagnosis of migraine, even if (as is often the case) patients only describe negative symptoms: one patient noted, for example, that a 'few weeks ago she had had a busy day rushing around seeing flats and was sitting on the bus when she noticed a silvery visual disturbance in her right visual field. About 20 minutes later she noticed some numbness of the right hand which slowly spread up her arm. Shortly afterwards she noticed that this numbness was affecting the right side of her lips and over the following 10–15 minutes it spread to involve the inside of the mouth, teeth and tongue on that side.' It is rare for sensory aura to affect both sides of the body simultaneously.

Sensory aura is disconcerting. Occasionally it will manifest as a feeling of heaviness on one side of the body, an odd discomfort, often described as being like the feeling of the arm going to sleep. This sensation of heaviness of one limb or one side of the body is not infrequently uncomfortable. More rarely there is actual pain in a limb or down one side of the body associated with the more typical tingling and numbness; this is perhaps distinct from the rare cases where migraine pain presents in the body (corpalgia) rather than the head. Some patients describe affected areas as feeling numb or detached from the rest of the body, as if the limb does not belong to them. Others describe affected areas as feeling hollow, stiff or cold. Even more rarely a combination of sensory disturbances can occur, as in the patient who described an attack beginning with a 'tight numb spasm feeling of the left side of the face and a freezing cold sensation in the left ear'. Sometimes the sensations are compared to ants crawling on the skin, or electric shocks in the limbs.

One celebrated but rare form of sensory aura causes disruption of the body image. Patients can describe a feeling that a part or the whole of their body feels abnormally large, or unusually small. This was christened 'Alice in Wonderland Syndrome' by the psychiatrist John Todd, in 1955. Todd speculated that Lewis Carroll had drawn on his own experiences of aura to inspire events in his novel, specifically the section when Alice first falls down the rabbit hole and consumes the cake and liquid that cause her to grow and shrink, respectively. Other commentators have speculated that the disappearance of the Cheshire Cat, leaving nothing but its smile, is a depiction of the effect of visual aura. Yet others dismiss this as a fanciful over-interpretation of the text.

Motor manifestations of aura are much rarer than visual or sensory symptoms, and are always invariably negative (that is, a loss of function rather than motor overactivity). Hemiplegic migraine, in which there is true one-sided weakness similar to that experienced by patients after a stroke, is fortunately rare, but striking. These attacks often lead (on the first occasion, at least) to a hospital admission and investigations aimed at establishing whether the sufferer has had a stroke, or an episode of inflammation within the brain or spinal cord. It is more common for migraine-associated weakness to be restricted to the face, causing drooping of one eyelid or of one side of the face. Positive motor symptoms are rare, but sufferers occasionally find one limb or side of the body becomes shaky or tremulous. Very rarely, patients nod during the aura phase. Motor aura typically lasts for hours before recovering, though in rare but well-documented cases the weakness can last for days, or even weeks or months. In these patients the other manifestations of aura can also persist for long periods, as in the following patient's experience:

> She woke up with a feeling of right-sided heaviness, predominantly affecting her leg. She found that she could not lift her leg up properly. This was associated with a general feeling of numbness, blankness and detachment from her surroundings which she describes as very similar to her usual migraine. Indeed she says that she constantly felt through this period that she was about to have a migraine. Her walking was affected for a couple of months in total though it eased off at that stage. Over the first couple of days of the event she had almost complete speech

arrest. Afterwards she started to feel distinctly better but she found that her thoughts were blocked. Once again things have improved but she feels that her speech is still not back to normal and that she has a tendency to stammer or stutter. Her leg symptoms recur for a day or two every fortnight. These attacks are preceded by a burning sensation in the left foot and then a pinching pain in the right leg.

It is easy to see why, in an era before detailed CT and MRI imaging was available to demonstrate that such patients had *not* suffered a stroke, this patient and others like her might have been wrongly diagnosed. It is also easy to see why, even if patients have had similar episodes in the past, there is a tendency to submit patients with hemiplegic migraine to repeated scans. If these are MRI scans, then there is no down-side other than the use of resources; but repeated exposure to the X-ray radiation required for CT scanning does increase the risk of developing a brain tumour. I have written letters for a number of my patients specifically asking Emergency Departments *not* to scan them unless they have good reason to believe they are suffering from a different attack to usual. Judgement can of course be difficult in such cases.

Speech may be affected by migraine aura; most commonly, patients experience expressive dysphasia – that is, the inability to say words or sentences, whilst retaining understanding of what is said. This can vary in severity, from slowing of thought to simple word-finding difficulties (for example, inability to get words out correctly), through problems with grammar (such as the inability to string a sentence together when talking on the telephone) to unintelligible speech or 'goobledigook', as one patient put it, and ultimately to a total inability to produce any speech whatsoever. If comprehension is affected – this is termed a receptive dysphasia – then sufferers may appear confused. If mild, this may manifest itself as a difficulty processing verbal information, in much the same way that, as mentioned above, patients may struggle to process visual information, to extract meaning from what they hear or see. At other times speech problems may relate more to articulation – patients become dysarthric rather than dysphasic. Speech may become slurred, leading the casual observer to conclude that the symptoms are due to overindulgence in alcohol. Just occasionally people will stutter during the aura phase.

Auras affecting smell and taste are extremely rare. In this, migraine differs from epilepsy, in which focal seizures of temporal lobe origin often cause patients to experience unusual smells or tastes. It is of course possible that the true prevalence of olfactory aura is underestimated, as patients with these symptoms are generally referred to ENT departments rather than neurologists or headache experts. The presence of other typical migraine symptoms, and the absence of any obvious nasal or sinus problems on scanning or direct observation, may ultimately suggest the diagnosis.

Migraine-related dizziness is very common, a significant proportion of sufferers reporting it. True vertigo – that is, the sense of movement of the world around you, or the sense that you are moving when you are not – is also frequently reported. It is not clear whether vertigo is truly an aura phenomenon or not. As outlined below, aura is thought to be a process mediated on the surface of the brain, in the cerebral cortex, and vertigo has traditionally been thought of as a process that arises from the connections between the inner ears and the base of the brain. However, in recent years it has become clear that there are areas of the cortex in which the vestibular (balance) system is represented, and so it is perhaps most likely that vertigo in migraine patients is a manifestation of aura. Attacks can be prolonged, lasting minutes to hours, or very brief, lasting seconds only. Vertigo can become disconcerting, as in the case of one patient whose illusion of self-movement developed into 'a sinking feeling that the room is rising around her'. Vertigo and dizziness are often associated with a sense of imbalance or incoordination, which may be exacerbated by sensory impairment or weakness. Some commentators distinguish migraine with vertigo as a specific condition – vestibular migraine – but in my view it is just one of the many variants of migraine with aura, and should be understood and treated as such.

More subtle disturbances of cerebral function are probably common, but it is difficult to distinguish the direct effects of the aura process from the indirect effects of how aura makes one feel. This may in turn be exacerbated if the non-headache features of migraine start in the aura phase; it is fairly common, for example, for sufferers to begin to experience light or noise sensitivity, or nausea, at this point. This can develop into a sense of imbalance or unease; some people may describe 'a sense of heightened awareness and sensitivity . . . and a sense of tingling all over'. Occasionally experiences more typically seen in the premonitory or prodromal phase may persist into, or begin within, aura; some people, for example, experience cravings for sweet foods at this point. Patients can feel disconnected from their environment, disorientated or tearful; some may develop 'a strange feeling, a vacant look'. Occasionally they may lose the ability to perform certain tasks: one nurse described to me how, during a migraine aura, she would hear the alarm of a blocked feeding pump but be unable to work out how to stop it; if she developed an attack whilst driving, she would come to a roundabout and be completely unable to work out what to do.

Rarely this may develop into a full-blown sense of anxiety, and even more rarely an overwhelming sense of impending doom (*angor animi*). Subsequent to an attack of aura while driving, one of my patients developed an intense fear of recurrence, leading to panic attacks and agoraphobia that lasted for sixteen years.

More frequently, people will describe feeling vaguely 'weird'. At its worst this can be as debilitating as pain or weakness, when difficulties with conversation, clumsiness, unsteadiness and memory impairment cause cognitive and emotional difficulties which adversely impact both upon work and home life. The emotional impact of aura can long outlast the actual attack. One patient experiences prolonged attacks during which she suffers bad nightmares: 'The dreams are always very disturbing because they are vivid and brightly coloured/patterned like mosaic pattern or like Aladdin's carpet, or sometimes I feel like I'm trapped in a moving castle or in a moving kaleidoscope which is quite scary.' Others find aura intruding upon the subconscious: 'Often my friends have commented that I doodle in class at university, and one friend this year noticed I usually only draw half of a face, usually just the left . . .'

What causes aura?

> According to the other and alternative explanation of the disease, the primary derangement is of the nerve-cells of the brain. Their function from time to time is disturbed in a peculiar manner, . . . The periodical derangement of function has been called . . . a 'nerve-storm.'
>
> William Gowers, *A Manual of Diseases of the Nervous System* (1886)[11]

Advances in the understanding of brain function in the nineteenth century revealed that the visual centres of the brain
were at the rear, in the occipital lobes. They were thought to
be connected to an area at the base of the brain called the
optic thalamus. The physician Edward Liveing hypothesised
that migraine was due to a 'nerve-storm' passing through this
part of the brain. His Cambridge colleague Peter Wallwork
Latham, in common with leading continental scientists, suggested instead that aura was due to constriction of the blood
supply to the visual area of the brain, and the succeeding
headache due to expansion of the same vessels, possibly mediated through the sympathetic nervous system. This vascular
theory was simple to understand and popular, and it was the
most widely held explanation for aura for over a hundred
years; but it had its obvious problems, as the influential British
neurologist William Gowers had pointed out from the beginning. Constriction of the blood vessels should restrict blood
supply to a particular area of the brain and stop that area of
the brain working. If this affected the visual area of the brain,
it should cause a loss of vision. The sparkling scintillations
characteristic of aura were difficult to explain, as was the
progression of symptoms across the visual fields. It was also
clear that in many cases headache started before aura had
completely resolved, a fact which could not be explained by
the vascular theory. The great American neurologist Harold
Wolff, who was the first to demonstrate how blood flow in

extracranial blood vessels changed during migraine head-ache (and how the effective migraine medication ergotamine impacted upon this process), struggled to explain the phe-nomena, only devoting eight pages to it, out of the over 600 pages that made up the first edition of his seminal mono-graph *Headache and Other Head Pain* (1948).

A century after Liveing, Latham and Gowers, writing in *Migraine: Clinical and Research Aspects*, a collection of presenta-tions on migraine published at a pivotal moment in 1987, the London neurologist Nat Blau commented in his introductory chapter ('The patient observed') that most of the widely rec-ognised characteristics of migraine aura (a term which Blau himself had done much to promote) remained unexplained. It was not known, Blau wrote, why the occipital cortex was so prone to the process, nor why sensory symptoms should affect the face and arm more than the leg, or why motor symptoms should be so rare. Blau pointed out that it was not possible to account for an enlarging, slowly moving scotoma with a scintillating edge on the basis of the constriction of cerebral arteries, citing the leading stroke expert, C. Miller Fisher, who had written that he had not encountered such a visual disturbance in thirty-five years of studying stroke and transient ischaemic attacks. Miller Fisher had also pointed out that to postulate that constriction of the blood vessels could cause altered sensation without motor symptoms, would require spasm of the small posterior branches of the middle cerebral artery in sequence, without involving the anterior branches of the same artery, a state of affairs he called 'inconceivable'. Blau agreed. Nonetheless, aura symptoms were so characteristic and widely experienced, that the combination of positive and negative features, and the progression of symptoms, were both encapsulated within the definition of migraine aura produced by the Classification Committee of the International Headache Society in the early 1980s, over a century after Airy's original diagram had been produced.

By the mid 1980s, however, a new theory of aura was starting to emerge. Later in the same collection of essays edited by Blau, there was an article by the Danish neurologists Martin Lauritzen and Jes Olesen, in which they presented the results of their studies of cerebral blood flow in migraine. It was known that as many as 50 per cent of patients who were prone to visual aura would have an attack after carotid angiography (that is, the injection of a radio-opaque dye into the carotid arteries, used to provide pictures of the blood vessels in the brain in an era before CT or MRI scanning – and still in some circumstances today). The Danes used this as an opportunity to study their patients' cerebral circulation in the initial phases of a migraine attack by injecting radioactive xenon-133 into the carotid arteries. They found that in their migraine patients this caused a decrease in regional cerebral flow that began in the posterior part of the brain and progressed anteriorly in a slow wave, independent of the territories that were supplied by the large cerebral arteries. This led them to conclude that this process was mediated by a primary disturbance of nerve cell function, rather than being primarily vascular. Lauritzen and Olesen further surmised that the phenomenon that underlay those changes was 'Leão's spreading depression': a neurophysiological phenomenon first described by the Argentinian neurophysiologist Aristides Leão in the 1940s, in which a wave of excitation spread slowly across the surface of the brain, followed by a longer period of inhibition, before normal function was restored.

By the 1980s, cortical spreading depression (CSD) – as Leão's spreading depression had become known – was recognised to be a relatively common response of the cerebral cortex to various noxious stimuli (it is seen as a consequence of bleeding on the surface of the brain, for example). Lauritzen and Olesen induced CSD in laboratory rats and studied cerebral blood flow following this, finding that the patterns of blood flow and the accompanying physiological responses of the blood vessels were essentially identical to the pattern that they saw in their human migraine patients. They theorised, therefore, that aura was the experience of CSD: a neural tsunami initiated in the posterior (visual) part of the brain, and progressing anteriorly with a constant speed of approximately 2–3 mm/min, and that it was the transient absence of nervous activity that caused reduced blood flow to the affected areas.

The possibility that aura was a primarily neural process, consisting of a wave of excitation and then inhibition, had been raised before, most notably by the visual physiologist Karl Lashley, who in 1940 published meticulous descriptions of his own visual aura. In 1958 the Canadian neurologist P. M. Milner proposed Leão's spreading depression as a candidate process by which such a wave could propagate across the surface of the brain (as Leão himself had done), but it was not until Lauritzen and Olesen published their regional blood flow studies that this theory started to gain credence in the wider headache community.

And it remains a theory. It is very difficult to demonstrate CSD itself in the human brain, except in extreme cases of brain damage due to bleeding on the surface of the brain. However, numerous research studies have confirmed Lauritzen and Olesen's original findings, and have replicated them by other means, such as functional MRI scanning. In addition, CSD provides an explanation for the other manifestations of aura: if it starts in the occipital lobes and spreads forward, it will first affect regions that deal with sensory information. Further forward are the areas of the brain that deal with language, motor function, emotion and so on. CSD therefore has the potential to affect any cerebral function. Why it has a particular predilection for the occipital lobes, and why in most people it fizzles out before it reaches other parts of the brain, are questions that remain, now as in 1987, largely unanswered.

Treatments: acute, preventive and lifestyle

What acute treatments are available for headaches?

> *The application of ether to the temples, washing the head with cold water, the cephalic snuff, noticed above [leaves of tobacco, one ounce; ditto of rosemary, six drachms; ditto of asarabacca, two drachms; white hellebore root, two drachms . . . well dried and reduced to a fine powder], a blister to the nape of the neck, keeping the feet warm by wearing flannel socks, attention to the state of the digestive organs, and avoiding full meals and spirituous or vinous liquors, with moderate exercise, will, generally speaking, prove highly beneficial in mitigating, if not effectually curing habitual or chronic headachs, from whatever cause they may arise . . .*
>
> Richard Reece, *A Practical Dictionary of Domestic Medicine* (1808)[12]

Headache treatment has three pillars: lifestyle modifications and trigger management; acute treatments, to take when a headache occurs; and preventive treatments or interventions, designed to reduce the frequency and intensity of headaches, shorten their duration, and make them easier to treat with acute medications. Most people who get headaches will not need or want to take regular treatment for them, and some people get headaches that are so mild that they will not want to take any treatment for them at all. Usually, however, it is desirable to have some form of acute treatment to take when a headache comes, ideally to get rid of it altogether, or at the very least to make it less severe, to shorten it in duration and to reduce any other symptoms that might come with it, so as to make things more manageable, and allow one to get on with the normal activities of daily life.

For most people with headaches, their first port of call is the local pharmacy, where they will be able to buy over-the-counter (OTC) painkillers. What is available varies to a degree from country to country. In the United Kingdom (as is the case for most of the world), the standard OTC options comprise paracetamol (acetaminophen), aspirin and the non-steroidal anti-inflammatories (NSAIDs), such as ibuprofen, and combinations of these medications with caffeine (which has been shown to improve both the absorption and effectiveness of painkillers). In the UK, unlike some other countries, it is also possible to buy OTC combination therapies that contain small doses of codeine, alongside paracetamol, some of which are specifically marketed for headache or migraine treatment.

When taking any of these medications (and indeed the same is true for prescribed painkilling medication), they will generally be most effective if taken early on in the course of the headache, and at a dose that is most likely to stop the headache in its tracks early on. As we have seen in the section on the physiological processes that occur in headaches, there is a window of opportunity early on when some of those processes are occurring in and around the extracranial blood vessels to which painkillers, once absorbed through the gut, can get quickly and in reasonable quantities. Once these early processes have run their course, headache physiology becomes more central (that is, within the brain itself), and painkillers become much less effective as they cannot, for the most part, cross the blood–brain barrier. Once headaches, particularly migraines, are set in, they become much more difficult to treat.

Most people, therefore, will start with paracetamol or ibuprofen. Whilst these are generally very safe and well tolerated medications, it is of course important to stress that anyone proposing to take any form of medication should check with their pharmacist and/or GP that it is safe and appropriate for them to do so.

If these medications are not working properly (that is, if they do not touch the headache at all, or they have such a minimal effect that it is as if they had not worked at all), then this would be a sensible time to seek advice from a pharmacist or GP. For most types of pain, the World Health Organization pain ladder indicates that if simple analgesics are not working, then the next step is to move up to weak opiates, such as the small dose of codeine that is contained in OTC combination medications. However, for headache disorders, this may not be the best step. Generally speaking, opiates are not good treatments for headache. If people do not respond to simple analgesics, then it is unlikely that the headache is simply a tension-type headache, and is most probably going to be a migraine, or possibly one of the other, much rarer, primary headache disorders. In these circumstances, the appropriate next step could be a prescription of triptan.

The triptans are acute headache medications, first developed by the pharmacologist Pat Humphrey and his team at Glaxo in Ware, Hertfordshire, in the 1980s. Humphrey believed that serotonin was central to migraine physiology, and his team searched for new drugs that could impact upon serotonin systems in the brain, and thereby treat migraines. Using the best validated migraine model available at the time, they came up with a number of candidate drugs, one of which eventually came through to market in 1990 as sumatriptan. This proved to be a highly effective migraine treatment, and much safer than the previous gold standard treatment, ergotamine. It is still common to speak to patients who were prescribed triptans in the early 1990s, and experienced them as game- or life-changing drugs, capable of treating migraines in a way that no previous migraine medications had been able to achieve. Over the following ten years a further six triptans were released to market, and all seven of these drugs remain available today. So successful have the triptans been, that it is only now, in the 2020s, that new generations of acute migraine treatments are finally making their way to market (these will be mentioned in the section on future directions on page 169).

Most GPs will prescribe sumatriptan 50 mg as a first-line treatment if patients do not respond to OTC painkillers. Sumatriptan is the longest-established and cheapest of the triptans. If the starting dose is not effective, it can be dou-bled to 100 mg, or an alternative method of delivery (via nasal spray or subcutaneous self-injection) can be consid-ered. Overall, response rates to treatment with the various different triptans are very similar, though some patients will respond better to one member of the class than others, and it is always worth trying two or three different triptans if there is an inadequate response to the first one that is tried. The subcutaneous 6 mg formulation of sumatriptan remains, more than thirty years after it was the first triptan to become widely available, the most effective acute treatment we possess for migraine and cluster headache.

A small proportion of patients with migraine (perhaps about 10 per cent) are genuinely triptan non-responders, but poor response to medication is more often due to inadequate dosing, or poor absorption. In this regard, it is almost always useful for patients with migraine to take a prokinetic anti-sickness tablet (domperidone, for example, if appropriate) alongside any painkiller. Migraine often causes the gut to slow down (gastroparesis), so any medication that can counter this process, and also reduce nausea (which is often a particularly unpleasant aspect of migraine attacks) is likely to be helpful.

In the author's opinion, opiates should only very rarely be used as acute treatments for headache disorders. There are a very small number of patients for whom they are the most appropriate option, but they should always be the treatment of last resort. The reason for this is that, partly because they are not especially effective headache treatments, they run the highest risk of engendering rebound headaches, and ultimately causing medication overuse headache, a topic that will be covered in the next section (see page 71).

Dr Mark Weatherall

What happens when people take too many painkillers?

'His squire tells me that he is plagued by blinding headache and oft quaffs the milk of the poppy as lesser men quaff ale.'

Qyburn on Gregor Clegane,
from George R. R. Martin, *A Feast for Crows* (2005)[13]

Is it possible to have too much of a good thing? Is it possible that taking too many painkillers can actually be a bad thing, and make headaches worse? The answer to those questions is, in some cases, yes. This has been understood for a long time. There are clear descriptions of the worsening of headaches due to overindulgence in analgesics dating back to medical encyclopedias published in the first two decades of the twentieth century. But the definitive evidence that taking too many painkillers could make headaches worse only really emerged around the turn of the twenty-first century, with landmark studies that showed that people who were given regular painkillers for reasons other than headache (arthritis, for example) could develop headaches *de novo*, or find that their pre-existing headaches became worse. This effect seemed to be largely confined to people with a personal or family history of migraine.

The concept of 'medication overuse headache' entered the headache literature at that time, and medication overuse has become increasingly widely recognised as a problem over the last two decades. Many general practitioners are aware of the importance of trying to ensure that their patients do not take too many painkillers, as this can over time make things worse. The key to the diagnosis of medication overuse headache is time; it is very important to realise that having medication overuse headache does not simply mean having a lot of headaches and taking a lot of painkillers. To make a formal diagnosis, one needs to demonstrate a steady worsening of headache over a period of medication overuse; this requires, at the very least, the keeping of a reasonably extensive longitudinal headache diary. In cases of medication overuse headache, one will typically see a steady upward trend in the number of headache days each month. If this happens, one needs to look carefully for other reasons why things might be getting worse; many of the potential problems that could be occurring are covered in the later sections that cover lifestyle triggers (see page 119). I have looked after patients whose diaries indicate that they routinely have between seventeen and twenty-one days of migraine each month, and take painkillers successfully for all of those headaches. Some months are better than others, some months are worse. These patients do not have medication overuse headache, even though they are taking painkillers more often than the International Classification of Headache Disorders' (ICHD's) recommended fifteen days per month for simple analgesics such as paracetamol, or ten days per month for triptans, opiates or barbiturates. The diary shows that the use of these painkillers is not actually making things worse over time. There is a risk that if these patients are incorrectly labelled as having problematic medication overuse, and told to stop taking painkillers altogether, the baby will be thrown out with the bathwater, and their condition will suffer.

In cases of medication overuse headache, one will typically see not only a steady increase in the frequency of headaches, but also a steady decrease in the response to the use of these painkillers. It is not uncommon for patients to report that they originally responded very well to their acute medication, but then over time find themselves having to take ever higher and more frequent doses to get the same benefit. Gradually, an episodic headache problem will evolve (or 'transform', as mentioned in an earlier chapter – see page 19) into a chronic one, with little or no response to acute treatments at all. When you ask patients in this situation why they continue to take painkillers at all, if they do not work, they will often answer that they are afraid to stop doing so, in case things get worse.

Paradoxically, stopping the painkillers may be the best thing that these patients can do. In a small but significant proportion of patients with medication overuse headache, simply stopping the painkillers will cause the headache to completely resolve; in these cases, the headache is being purely and solely driven by the rebound pain resulting from the wearing-off of the previous dose. In a study that I undertook early on in my career as a consultant, I found that about 20 per cent of people in this situation experienced a complete or near-complete resolution of their headache when they stopped taking painkillers. A more common outcome was that things improved, with headaches becoming less frequent or more manageable; they often found that other treatments that I gave them afterwards (preventive medication, for the most part) worked better than they had before. This improvement of response to treatment once medication overuse has been addressed has been demonstrated in a number of trials over the years; the first such study was published by the team at the Danish Headache Centre over two decades ago.

Over time, the diagnostic criteria for medication overuse headache have become increasingly specific about the maximum frequency at which different painkillers should be taken. A consensus has emerged around the figures now embedded in the ICHD (as mentioned above: fifteen days per month for simple analgesics; ten days per month for triptans, opiates or barbiturates). Some authorities set even more strict limits than this. I find that a reasonable rule of thumb is that people should not find themselves needing to take painkillers on more than a couple of days a week, and that if they routinely have to do so, then preventive treatments and a period of medication withdrawal should be considered.

This is an area where keeping a headache diary can be helpful. Without keeping contemporary records, it is easy to downplay analgesic consumption. Sometimes it is only when someone writes everything down that they realise how dependent they have become on their daily dose of Co-codamol, or sumatriptan. Studies have shown that non-steroidal anti-inflammatories (such as ibuprofen) are less likely to cause medication overuse, and indeed in small quantities they may actually make it less likely that migraine will transform from an episodic into a chronic form.

What, then, is the best way of treating medication overuse headache? It is very easy to simply say, 'You must stop taking your painkillers,' but this naturally leads to a follow-up question: 'What do I do then, when I have a headache?' Persuading people not to take painkillers is generally easier if those painkillers do not work. In other cases, the conversation is more difficult, and it is important to explain the rationale behind the restriction in the use of painkillers, and to have a follow-on plan of what to do if things do not improve. There are varying views on how best to approach this. The traditional 'European' view was that patients should undergo complete medication withdrawal for a period of up to two months; at the end of that time some consideration could be given to the use of preventive medication if necessary. The 'American' viewpoint was that it was a violation of a person's inalienable rights to deprive them of all medication, and according to this view it was better to start preventive medication and then attempt medication withdrawal, rather than the other way around. The latter approach has come to predominate over recent years as evidence has mounted that it is more likely to work overall. However the 'withdrawal first, preventive later' approach continues to offer the potential advantage that, as mentioned above, a reasonable proportion of people will improve so much that they do not need to go on to preventive treatment. There is no right answer here; treating medication overuse is an art, requiring an open and honest conversation between a patient and their medical practitioner, an early agreed follow-up to review progress and alter treatment if necessary, and a plan about how to manage any other symptoms that appear during the process of medication withdrawal.

It is probably inadvisable to attempt to go 'cold turkey' if one is taking strong opiates (such as codeine phosphate or tramadol) or barbiturates, and/or if there are significant medical or psychiatric co-morbidities (such as severe anxiety or depression). Where people come off weaker opiates, experiences such as palpitations, sweating and difficulty sleeping are common, and can be prepared for and treated, if necessary. Some clinical trials have shown that giving patients a short course of a few days' treatment with oral steroids can be helpful in getting them over the initial rebound worsening of headache that is often experienced. When steroids were first introduced into medicine in the 1950s, they were widely regarded as a miracle treatment as they were helpful for many conditions for which there had previously been nothing to be done. Over the following decades, people threw steroids at most medical problems for which they did not have a solution; one of these problems was persistent or refractory headache. As noted in a later chapter (see page 110), short courses of steroids have found a place as a transitional treatment for cluster headache. But steroids will non-specifically settle down most types of headache, in perhaps 30 to 50 per cent of cases. They are not a viable long-term treatment option because of their side effects (increased blood pressure, increased blood sugar, bone thinning, muscle weakness and so on), but short courses are usually tolerated well, and can be a helpful adjuvant option in getting patients off their painkillers. Steroids commonly cause stomach irritation and insomnia, and are best taken in the morning with breakfast. Patients should also be warned of a temporary increased susceptibility to infection, and of the rare side effects of euphoria or avascular necrosis (an interruption to the blood supply of the bones). Doctors and patients alike are often wary of steroids, but their judicious employment in this scenario can be very beneficial.

Some authorities approach the problem in two stages by initially switching patients from regular opiate or triptan use to the regular use of an anti-inflammatory such as naproxen. This risks simply substituting one problem for another, but as mentioned above the anti-inflammatories are less likely to drive headaches in the way that other analgesics do, and the second step of stopping them is likely to be associated with fewer and more manageable withdrawal effects.

Epidemiological studies undertaken in the early 2000s showed that about 2 to 3 per cent of the population in western societies experience daily headaches, and about half of these people are taking painkillers on a daily basis. Basic research shows that people with chronic migraine and medication overuse have increased levels of CGRP, changes in their endocannabinoids (the body's own cannabis-like substances that are believed to be intimately involved in pain processing, inflammation and other neural processes), and alterations in their endogenous pain control systems. Medication overuse causes persistent central sensitisation, which leads to increased levels of pain induced by exposure to normal levels of light, noise and touch. Functional imaging studies show multiple changes in the brain activity in people taking regular painkillers; fortunately, these changes largely reverse when patients undergo successful medication withdrawal.

The more widespread acknowledgement of the importance of recognising and treating medication overuse has been one of the successes of headache education over the last two decades. Few general practitioners are unaware of the problems that can arise from taking too many painkillers, and many pharmacies now have electronic systems in place to flag up people taking painkillers regularly, and call them for review. As outlined above, however, guiding people through medication overuse requires clinical judgement and a willingness and ability to follow up people at intervals throughout the process. This process requires the close attention of the healthcare professional, and tenacity from the patient, but successful outcomes are rewarding for both parties.

The principles of preventive treatment of headaches

An ounce of prevention is worth a pound of cure.
Benjamin Franklin, 1736[14]

Most people with headaches will not need to take regular medication, or have other regular interventions for their headaches. They will manage them successfully with painkillers and other medications taken at the time of the attacks. In some cases, however, attacks come so frequently that acute painkillers either start to become less effective, or are being taken so frequently that patients run the risk of developing headaches as a consequence of taking painkillers too often (medication overuse headache – see previous section, 'What happens when people take too many painkillers?'). In these circumstances, some form of regular preventive treatment may be appropriate. Such treatment might also be considered in the rarer circumstances where patients do not respond to acute painkillers at all, or cannot take them because of allergies or other medication conditions that make it inadvisable for them to do so.

Some people worry that starting regular medication for headaches means that they are going to be on treatment for the rest of their lives, but that is extremely unlikely to be the case. Headache disorders rise and fall in people's lives. People with headaches often have spells when they are very active, and other periods when everything calms down; in the majority of cases, headaches will eventually settle down altogether. It is just not possible to predict with any exactness or certainty when this will happen. Preventive treatment is therefore best regarded as an intervention with the aim of improving headache control and thereby quality of life, at those points where headaches become so active and/or difficult to treat, that they are impacting upon everyday well-being (as outlined in the section that discusses what makes headaches a disease rather than just a normal lived experience – see page 22).

The main principle of preventive treatment is therefore that it should be considered when headaches are so frequent or severe that they are impacting on people's quality of life (there is no set frequency or severity at which this kicks in, as this must always be judged in the context of the individual's personal preferences and circumstances). Options for preventive treatment should be discussed with patients, and the choice of treatment based on a consideration of the efficacy of treatment, while also taking into account other factors such as the side-effect profile of any proposed treatment (which in some cases may make particular options inadvisable, for example, avoiding beta-blockers in people with an active history of asthma or other chronic airways disease). Logistical or administrative restrictions may affect the availability of some options, particularly if treatment is being delivered through the NHS. Patient preference should, as always, be taken into account if it is practicable to do so.

Before starting preventive medication, patients should be encouraged to keep a headache diary. This does not need to be a particularly detailed affair, particularly if it is primarily being used for the purpose of assessing response to treatment, but it should at least contain basic information on the frequency and severity of headache: a daily score of 0–10, where 0 is no pain at all, and 10 is the worst imaginable pain, is commonly used; alternatively, patients can simply record each day whether their pain has been 'mild', 'moderate' or 'severe', or if they have been pain-free. This diary should be reviewed with the patient at intervals to judge the effectiveness or otherwise of treatment.

Oral preventive treatments should be started at a low dose, and built up steadily over time. The question is always whether the positive effects of treatment will kick in before any side effects do. It is useful for patients and the prescribing doctor to have a clear plan from the outset of what the target dose of any oral preventive medication should be. As the doses of oral preventive treatments are steadily increased, most patients will start to get a sense of whether they are going to be helpful, though the maximum benefit may not accrue until the patient reaches the target or maximum tolerated dose. Again, there is no set timescale for this process, nor is there any set length of time for which treatment should be taken before deciding that it is ineffective, but it is probably fair to say that if patients have built up an oral treatment up to a maximum tolerated or target dose, and have derived no benefit from it after staying on that dose for six to eight weeks, then it is extremely unlikely that it is suddenly going to start working at that point, and it is probably time to move on.

In the headache world, the usual practice is monotherapy – that is, one preventive treatment at a time. Traditionally prevention has been started with oral medication, before moving on to other interventions or treatment options, and for the most part this remains standard practice. In the following sections I will outline some of the oral preventives that are typically used to prevent tension-type headaches, migraines and cluster headaches, as well as outpatient interventions such as nerve blocks and Botox, and some of the newer treatments, for example the CGRP monoclonal antibodies. There is also a section on non-invasive neuromodulation, which has had a small but interesting role in the treatment of migraine and cluster headache in recent years.

One area that I do not cover in detail is the psychological therapies that have been shown to be potentially effective in treating headaches. The interventions most commonly studied in this area are relaxation training, cognitive behavioural therapy (including mindfulness) and biofeedback. Studies generally indicate a modest benefit from such therapies. If they are delivered face-to-face, the greater the amount of contact time with a therapist, the greater the effect. Few prospective clinical trials of these techniques have been undertaken, and it is an area ripe for further research, and for the development of online resources that will allow headache sufferers to harness some of the benefits of these approaches without direct recourse to scarce psychological personnel.

Finally, there is the question of how long preventive treatment should be continued, if it is successful. In most cases people will have started preventive treatment because of very active or severe headaches. Headache disorders do have a momentum, in general, and if this momentum can be slowed down, then many patients will find that, if they can achieve good control of their headaches for a reasonable length of time (perhaps six to twelve months in most cases), they can then start to come off preventive medication without the headaches immediately bouncing back again; it is helpful to set this as an expectation from the beginning, particularly when using novel or expensive therapies. It is easy for people to become psychologically dependent upon effective therapies, and wish to continue them long after they are biologically no longer necessary. I have struggled for many years to persuade my aged Columbian mother that she no longer needs to take the tiny (almost homeopathic) dose of propranolol that she was put on many years ago to prevent her migraines. At the time of writing, I have not yet succeeded in doing so.

What oral preventive treatments are available?

Do not undervalue the headache. While it is at its sharpest it seems a bad investment; but when relief begins, the unexpired remainder is worth $4 a minute.

Mark Twain, *Following the Equator*, 1897[15]

There are no definitive rules about when to use preventive medication, or which option is the best for any individual person. Modern guidelines such as the British Association for the Study of Headache's headache management system present clinicians and their patients with a series of options for which there is evidence derived from properly conducted clinical trials. These medications may reduce the intensity and frequency of headaches for some people, but there are no panaceas or magic bullets; not everything works for everybody.

The principles of preventive treatment have been set out in the previous section. In this section I will present some basic details of the medications and classes of oral medications that are most commonly used to prevent headaches, particularly but not exclusively migraine. The order that I present them is, broadly speaking, a 'batting order' that one might consider, but as will become apparent, certain medications may be inappropriate for, and contraindicated in certain patients. Ultimately, decisions about treatment need to be made in discussion with the prescribing clinician, taking into account the patient's personal medical history and preferences.

Amitriptyline and the other tricyclic antidepressants

The first clinical trial of amitriptyline as a preventive treatment for migraine was published in 1969. It was a very small trial, even by the standards of the day, and has never been repeated, although amitriptyline has since been put up against other preventive treatments in what are called 'non-inferiority' trials. Tricyclic antidepressants were introduced for their original purpose in the 1950s and 1960s, and patients were typically given high doses, often to a point where they were very sedated by them. They are still available for use as antidepressants, though they have perhaps been out-competed by modern drugs such as fluoxetine (Prozac) and other medications that impact on serotonin metabolism (interestingly, trials clearly show that these medications do not reliably reduce headaches). For pain, and headache, they remain commonly used and often effective options, typically starting at much smaller doses than would have been used in the past. For headaches, for example, one would usually start with the smallest possible dose of amitriptyline (10 mg) and build up steadily in 10–25 mg steps, trying to find a 'sweet spot' at which a positive benefit is gained without significant side effects kicking in, and making further up-titration of the dose inadvisable or impossible.

The common side effects of the tricyclics are drowsiness, dry eyes and dry mouth. They are best taken once a day, in the evening, usually about ten to twelve hours before the patient wants to get up in the morning. There is no specific maximum dose, other than that recommended in the British National Formulary, so long as the patient tolerates it, but if it has not proved helpful by the time the patient is taking between 50 and 100 mg at night, it is unlikely that it will suddenly kick in at a higher level.

Some clinicians favour other members of the tricyclic family, such as nortriptyline or dosulepin, on the basis that they may sometimes be better tolerated. It is certainly worth considering switching to an alternative tricyclic if amitriptyline seems to be helpful but not being tolerated particularly well. Whilst selective serotonin reuptake inhibitors (SSRIs) such as fluoxetine, sertraline and citalopram do not reduce migraines, the related class of selective serotonin and noradrenalin reuptake inhibitors (SNRIs), such as venlafaxine, may be helpful and are worth considering in cases where migraine is co-morbid with depression or anxiety. The most old-fashioned antidepressants of all – the monoamine oxidase inhibitors – used to be taken as migraine preventives of last resort, but are hardly ever prescribed nowadays, not least because of the danger of provoking a hypertensive crisis if a strict dietary regime is not adhered to while taking them.

Beta-blockers

The other standard first-line medication in the UK, of which most general practitioners will be aware and use to reduce migraines specifically, are beta-blockers. These are drugs that were first devised to reduce high blood pressure, but they are in a sense the 'Swiss Army penknives' of medicine, in that they not only reduce blood pressure and settle high or irregular heart rates, but they also (independently) improve heart failure and reduce migraine, tremor, intra-ocular pressure (given topically to the eyes of patients with glaucoma), thyrotoxicosis, and anxiety. Positive trials of a number of beta-blockers were carried out and published in the 1970s and 1980s. The most commonly used member of the class for migraine is propranolol, followed by atenolol, metoprolol, nadolol and bisoprolol. The advantage of propranolol is that it can be started at a very tiny dose (10 mg), which can then be built up slowly to a point where it is being taken two or three times a day, according to tolerability and effect. There is a once-daily slow release formulation of propranolol, which may be easier to remember to take. The original trials of propranolol were done at a dose of 240 mg a day, but many people will find it effective at much lower doses. The commonest side effects of beta-blockers are light-headedness, dizziness, cold extremities, odd dreams, decreased libido and impairment of exercise tolerance. As beta-blockers keep the pulse rate controlled, some patients find it difficult to exert themselves or exercise whilst taking these medications; everything feels slowed down or difficult, almost as if one is constantly 'wading through treacle'. It is important not to underestimate how debilitating these side effects, however vague, can become.

It is said (without much convincing supporting evidence, to be fair) that other beta-blockers may be better tolerated. Atenolol, for example, is not thought to cross the blood–brain barrier as effectively as propranolol, and may therefore cause fewer brain-related adverse effects, such as fatigue. Beta-blockers with partial agonist properties (that is, drugs that both block and stimulate the body's beta-adrenoreceptors), which are sometimes used by cardiologists, are not effective for migraine; these include carvedilol, nebivolol and celiprolol.

Other blood pressure medications

In the early 2000s, a headache research group in Norway was told by a couple of their patients that their headaches had improved after they had been put on what was then a relatively new blood pressure medication called candesartan. Clinical trials of this medication, published in 2003 and 2013, demonstrated its effectiveness in reducing migraine, and it has become increasingly widely used for this purpose over the last decade. Like any blood pressure medication, it can cause light-headedness and dizziness. It can also sometimes cause a degree of gastric irritation, though this is rarely bad enough to stop treatment. The original trials were done at a dose of 16 mg, with the patients being put straight on to this dose (I like to think they were sturdy Viking types impervious to side effects), but it is more typically the case that one would start at 4–8 mg and work steadily up to this level. There is some evidence that the frequency and intensity of migraines can be reduced by taking one of the other members of this class of medication (telmisartan) as well as a related blood pressure medication, lisinopril (which is an ACE inhibitor), though these are rarely used in everyday practice.

An interesting insight into the potential mechanism of action (or at least, a potential location of action) of candesartan and related drugs has emerged, unexpectedly, out of the work done on the SARS-Cov-2 virus, the cause of the Covid-19 pandemic. It was discovered very early on in the pandemic that the virus enters host cells in the human body by binding to angiotensin converting enzyme-2 (ACE2), which is expressed on cell surfaces in a number of different parts of the body. This includes the heart, the kidneys, the lungs, and – as it turned out – several brain tissues. One such was the olfactory nerves, the ends of which poke out in the nasal passages, allowing receptors to bind to circulating substances in those passages and generate the experience of smell and taste. Damage to those nerves caused by the entry of SARS-Cov-2 explains the loss of smell and taste so characteristic of the first wave of Covid-19 infections in 2020. It turns out, however, that ACE2 is also found on the surface of cells in the trigeminal ganglion; this is a relay station in the feedback loop between the brain and the blood vessels that line the membranes of the brain that runs hot at the start of a migraine attack. This was not known before the upsurge in interest in ACE2 that was driven by the need to understand the way in which the SARS-Cov-2 virus works. It is at least possible that drugs like candesartan work by binding to ACE2 in the trigeminal ganglion, and thereby impeding the early wind-up of signals through that ganglion that characterises the beginning of a migraine attack.

Anticonvulsants

The relationship between headaches and epilepsy has been contentiously debated since at least the 1870s. Over time it has become clear that the pathophysiological processes that underpin epileptic seizures, and migraine pain and auras, are fundamentally different, but it is the case that some drugs may damp down both processes. Not all epilepsy drugs work for migraine, though most of them have been put through clinical trials at some point. Looking back in the historical literature, one finds early epilepsy drugs such as bromide and phenobarbitone being touted as remedies for headache as far back as the start of the twentieth century, but it was not really until the 1980s, when clinical trials of sodium valproate showed it to be an effective migraine preventive, that anticonvulsants started to enter routine headache practice.

In the twenty-first century, however, the use of sodium valproate to treat migraine has largely been restricted to the treatment of men, or post-menopausal women, as evidence has emerged of a high potential for this drug to cause adverse effects on fetal development, and subsequent cognitive development in infancy, of children exposed to it *in utero*. Significant efforts are being made within the neurological community to minimise its use in women of childbearing age. Sodium valproate is however a very effective drug for migraine, and is probably underutilised in those patient populations for whom it would be an appropriate option. Like all anticonvulsants, sodium valproate can make people a little drowsy, dizzy or shaky. It can stimulate the appetite, causing people to put on weight if they are not careful about what they eat. Very rarely it can cause inflammation of the liver or pancreas, or a rash, and anyone starting the medication should always be warned about this and advised to seek medical attention if anything like this occurs. Sodium valproate can be given most conveniently as a once-daily slow-release formulation, usually in the evening, typically started at a dose of 200–500 mg at night, increased in migraine as high as 1200–1500 mg at night if necessary and tolerated.

The other anticonvulsant for which there is high-quality evidence for benefit in migraine (and chronic migraine) is topiramate. This was introduced as an epilepsy drug in the 1990s, and the company behind it invested heavily in migraine trials, seeking (successfully) to obtain an FDA licence for this indication in the USA. I tell my patients that topiramate is like Marmite – that they will either love it or hate it. It can be a very effective treatment, and for patients who are badly affected by chronic migraine, it has the requisite 'oomph' to be a gamechanger for some of them. Unfortunately, many people do not get on with it at all well. In addition to the potential adverse effects common to all epilepsy drugs, mentioned above, topiramate often causes tingling in the fingers, brain fog and speech arrest; this last condition exacerbates people's entirely normal propensity to get halfway through a sentence and suddenly find themselves completely unable to find the right word for something. This is of course a normal experience – everyone knows how frustrating it can be – but it does seem to be very specifically much worse for people who take topiramate, and for those people who earn a living by speaking fluently (barristers, teachers, newsreaders and so on), such an apparently innocuous side effect can in fact be extremely damaging. Topiramate can also raise intraocular pressure and cause glaucoma, create kidney stones and (fortunately rarely) cause very low mood or intrusive unpleasant thoughts. Another common side effect is appetite suppression, leading to weight loss. In modern society this is usually quite a good thing, but I have had a few patients over the years who cannot stop losing weight on topiramate, and the drug had to be stopped when their weight fell to dangerously low levels. The original clinical trials tested the overall benefit of the drug at various levels, and the 'Goldilocks dose' (that is, the one that fell between too small a dose that was ineffective, and too large a dose that was not generally tolerated) was 50 mg twice a day.

Several other epilepsy drugs have been the subject of clinical trials in migraine, and some have shown promising results, but none are widely used in everyday practice. Gabapentin, which is pretty much useless for epilepsy, but has some utility in patients with neuropathic (nerve) pain, used to be quite widely prescribed as a migraine preventive, until it was shown (in the US courts) that important data had been left out of the published trials. Once this additional data was added back in, the apparently positive effect of gabapentin largely disappeared. Some clinicians favour the use of other epilepsy drugs such as pregabalin or lamotrigine, but there is no good-quality evidence to support this. There is a reasonably convincing trial that shows that levetiracetam (perhaps the most widely used of the modern first-line drugs for epilepsy, because of its undoubted efficacy and tolerability) can be helpful in migraine, but this has not yet translated into widespread use for this indication.

Pizotifen

Pizotifen holds the distinction of being the migraine preventive in longest continuous use since the publication of the original clinical trial demonstrating its effectiveness (which appeared in 1965). The drug has a number of properties (it is, for example, an antihistamine), but its effect in migraine probably relates to its impact on serotonin metabolism. It was one of a set of drugs released in the 1960s that influenced serotonin levels in the brain and body. The others have either been withdrawn because they were no longer felt to be commercially profitable (methysergide), or have fallen into disuse because of lack of efficacy (cyproheptadine). Pizotifen, however, still warrants a place in the preventive pharmacopoeia because it works in a completely different way to any of the other options that we have, and can sometimes work surprisingly well when everything else has failed. It is commonly used in children. Its effectiveness can be limited by drowsiness, increased appetite, or vivid dreams.

Flunarizine

Flunarizine is one of the most widely used migraine preventives around the world. If you go to a migraine clinic in mainland Europe, Asia or South America, you are as likely to be prescribed this drug as you would be to come away from a clinic in the UK with a prescription for amitriptyline or propranolol. It is a calcium channel-blocker, originating as a blood pressure drug, but not generally used for this purpose. It is said to be the most effective drug for the more severe forms of migraine with aura. It is pretty much the only preventive medication that has been trialled in vestibular migraine, and is widely regarded as the drug of choice for patients with prolonged aura or hemiplegic migraine. It has an unusually long half-life (eighteen days), so for the most part patients do not need to increase the dose; they just need to keep taking it, and it will build up in their system over eight to twelve weeks.

Most patients tolerate flunarizine well, though it can cause dizziness and constipation (these side effects are common to all calcium channel-blockers, including verapamil, which is covered in the section on treating cluster headache (see page 12)), and very rarely can cause lowering of mood, or the development of muscle stiffness and slowness in a fashion that resembles the onset of Parkinson's disease. All of these side effects are reversible, though again because of the long half-life, they may take some time to wear off. Flunarizine is not in the British National Formulary, but it is available on prescription on what is called a 'named patient' basis, and is certainly a drug that should be offered in specialist headache centres to selected patient populations.

How does Botox help headaches?

'People say I look so happy – and I say, "That's the Botox."'
Dolly Parton (2021)[16]

Like many other headache treatments in common use, the fact that Botox could help headaches was discovered by accident. Botulinum toxin is one of the most dangerous substances known to mankind. In the wrong doses and the wrong places, it can cause muscle paralysis, respiratory failure and death. The last outbreak of botulism in the United Kingdom occurred in the 1990s, caused by the consumption of mushrooms that had not been cleaned and stored properly. Around this time, the toxin was starting to be used in medical practice. The first description of its use in a highly diluted form (Oculinum) to cause controlled amounts of muscle weakness was in work carried out by the ophthalmologist Alan Scott, as a treatment for squint caused by overactive ocular muscles. Approval for this research was granted in 1978, and the drug, by then renamed Botox, was given general approval by the FDA in the USA for use in squint and eyelid spasm in 1989. Some clever Canadian plastic surgeons quickly realised that Botox could be used for cosmetic purposes, and the first FDA approval for cosmetic treatment (specifically, of frown lines) was granted three years later, and a huge industry was born.

In the mid 1990s a small number of case reports were published, detailing the positive impact of Botox treatment given for cosmetic reasons, or for eyelid spasm, on the headaches previously experienced by those patients. Allergan, the company who owned Botox at the time, quickly picked up on these reports and immediately set up a series of clinical trials to see if they could demonstrate a consistent, clinically meaningful effect on headache following treatment with Botox. In the initial trials, some patients did very well, but the overall effect was not sufficient. Over time, additional injections at the back of the head and in the neck were added to the original protocol of injections in the forehead and temples. When the trials were then focused in upon those patients with the most severe, chronic form of migraine (that is, people having headaches more than fifteen days each month, at least half of which were full-blown migraines), statistically and clinically significant results started to emerge.

This process culminated in the two large-scale PREEMPT trials, undertaken in the USA and published in 2008. In these trials, patients with chronic migraine were given two sets of Botox injections, three months apart. Each set comprised thirty-one to thirty-nine individual injections of five units of Botox, thirty-one of which were given in standard positions, to the procerus, corrugator, frontalis, temporalis and occipitalis muscles over the skull, and to the cervical paraspinal and trapezius muscles in the neck. Clinicians were allowed to give patients up to a further eight injections in what was termed a 'follow-the-pain' manner (in other words, where patients felt the worst head pain). When the trial was published, it didn't seem to be the case that the additional injections had made much of a difference. Overall, however, the results were very impressive. Before treatment, patients on average had had twenty headache days each month. This fell by 50 per cent after two sets of Botox. Patients who had received placebo injections had also noticed a reduction in their headache frequency, but not to the same extent. It was on this basis that a licence was granted in 2010 in the USA and UK for the use of Botox to treat chronic migraine.

In the real world, it is perhaps most helpful to divide the response to Botox into three categories. Firstly you have what the Americans call 'super-responders'. These people find that Botox very significantly reduces, and in some cases almost completely turns off, their migraines. Up to one-third of patients can respond in this way. Another one-third of patients will get some benefit from Botox, in that it reduces the intensity and/or frequency of their attacks. In these patients, repeated treatments can sometimes bring cumulative benefits over a length of time. The final third of patients derive little or no benefit from Botox. It is always worth giving these patients a second chance with Botox, as in a small proportion (probably no more than 10 per cent) the second treatment will work where the first did not.

Botox given for chronic migraine has proved to be very safe and well tolerated over the years. The commonest significant side effect is cosmetic. About one in twenty patients develop a slight drooping of an eyelid, or furrowing of the eyebrows. This is due to the effect of Botox on the muscles of the forehead, and is not a permanent effect. If these patients have responded positively to the treatment, then small adjustments can be made to the position of future injections to reduce the chances of a recurrence of these cosmetic effects. Sometimes people will find the injections quite sore (especially if they have a bad migraine at the time they are given) or will develop flu-like symptoms in the first twenty-four hours, but more serious side effects are almost unheard of. Whenever I give patients Botox for the first time, I always counsel them to seek medical attention immediately should they experience any difficulties speaking, swallowing or breathing. I am able to reassure them, however, that there are no reports of patients ever experiencing these types of problem after being given Botox as per the PREEMPT protocol.

At the time of its introduction in 2010–12, Botox was very much a game-changer in the treatment of people with previously intractable migraine. It is not, and never will be a panacea, but many patients find it very effective, and even with the advent of other effective new options for migraine treatment, such as the CGRP monoclonal antibodies, there are a set of patients for whom Botox works better than anything else, and allows them to get on with their lives, largely free of their previous debilitating headaches.

Despite a quarter of a century of research and clinical practice, we do not fully understand exactly how Botox works for migraine. It is not the effect on the motor nerves that is harnessed in the treatment of muscle overactivity, and in cosmetic procedures. It is likely to be an effect mediated through the sensory nerves. Experiments done with American medical students (who will do anything for money) show that injecting Botox into the scalp reduces the pain brought on by rubbing chilli powder into the skin. It is likely that Botox modulates the way that sensory nerves send information back in to the TCC (the part of the brain that generates headaches) and thereby damps down activity in that region.

This hypothesis also explains why greater occipital nerve blocks – injections of local anaesthetic + / − steroid into the skin overlying the points at which these nerves curve round the base of the skull and dive through the muscle layers in the neck on their way to the second and third cervical nerve roots – can be helpful (albeit temporarily, for days or a few weeks) for settling down migraine, cluster headache and other primary headache disorders. These injections are simple, often effective, and very safe, the worst reported side effect being localized hair loss at the injection site (this has happened to fewer than 1 in 1000 of the patients on whom I have performed this treatment).

What are CGRP monoclonal antibodies?

Medicine is a tyranny of facts. Migraine is no exception.
Nat Blau, *Migraine –*
Clinical and Research Aspects (1987)[17]

As outlined in the section on CGRP (see page 35), much of the emphasis in basic and pharmaceutical migraine science over the last twenty-five years has been on finding treatments that will impact upon the release of CGRP. The four existing CGRP monoclonal antibodies (mAbs) that have been put through properly conducted clinical trials are a class of drugs that selectively and specifically attach themselves to CGRP or its receptor, and block its action. They are preventive treatments, the idea being to mop up CGRP *before* it enables the migraine pathways to become so active that people experience pain and other migraine symptoms. The initial clinical trials of the mAbs were published between 2014 and 2016, and the full Phase III trials between 2018 and 2020. Licensing in the USA and Europe soon followed. Four drugs have been approved (with certain stipulations and restrictions) by NICE for use in the NHS in England and Wales, and by the Scottish Medicines Consortium for use in the NHS in Scotland.

One of the mAbs (erenumab) targets the CGRP receptor, while the others bind to the molecule itself. This does not seem to make much of a difference to the overall effectiveness of the treatment. Indeed the results of the clinical trials are virtually identical across the board, although eptizenumab (which is delivered by an infusion given every twelve weeks) does have slightly higher response rates overall, but this is mainly due to the fact that the placebo response to this treatment is higher than it is for the other three mAbs (which are given by patients to themselves by subcutaneous injection, usually once every four weeks). The average response rate for patients with episodic migraine (that is, a baseline of four to fourteen migraine days each month) is of the order of three to four fewer days per month, and in chronic migraine (more than fifteen migraine days each month) of six to eight fewer days per month. Initially this may not sound hugely impressive, but in the case of chronic migraine in particular, this level of reduction of migraine is often enough to make a significant difference to people's quality of life.

It is also important to understand that the *average* response is made up of a wide variety of levels of improvement. When discussing the likelihood or otherwise of these medications being helpful, I generally present patients with the 50 per cent and 75 per cent response rates – that is, the proportion of those patients who after taking these treatments for three months experience a reduction in migraine days of more than 50 per cent, or more than 75 per cent (the latter group being the equivalent of the Botox 'super-responders').

In patients with chronic migraine, who should be the most refractory to treatment, the 50 per cent response rate is about 40 to 50 per cent, which compares very favourably with the response rates seen after Botox injections, or when treated with medications such as topiramate. When one factors in the extreme positive tolerability and (thus far) safety profile of these drugs, they are proving to be really helpful options for people struggling with the very worst type of primary headache disorders.

In terms of side effects, the commonest 'real world' problem is constipation, something which wasn't immediately obvious from the original clinical trials, but which rapidly became apparent when the drugs moved into general clinical practice. This has in a very tiny number of patients become bad enough to require hospitalisation. Some patients experience skin reactions at the injection sites, but these are rarely sufficiently bad to require a cessation or change in treatment. Other commonly reported effects are fatigue and a runny nose, but these are seen no more commonly than in the placebo arms of the original trials.

CGRP is widely distributed within the body, and is postulated to have more generalised actions in pain processing, as well as roles in the gastrointestinal tract, wound healing and so on. The mAbs remain relatively new drugs, and it is important for clinicians, and patients, to be watchful for unexpected problems and more subtle longer-term side effects. A few cases of newly raised blood pressure have been reported in patients taking erenumab in the USA, and there have been a small number of cases of worsening of Raynaud's phenomenon or autoimmune diseases in patients on one or other of the mAbs. Caution should be exercised in using these treatments in people who have these problems alongside migraine. There is as yet only one report in the literature of a serious neurological event in close temporal proximity to the use of a CGRP mAb, this being a woman who suffered a stroke shortly after her first dose of a mAb. Given the widespread and rapid take-up of these drugs (particularly in the USA, where tens of thousands of patients are now using them), the lack of further cases of this nature is cautiously reassuring.

Migraine does of course rise and fall in people's lives, and if one can take the momentum out of migraine networks within the brain by use of effective preventive treatments, then it is often the case that people will not need to stay on that treatment for extended periods. As a headache community in the UK, we have encouraged clinicians and patients to consider treatment pauses at intervals (perhaps every twelve to eighteen months), to assess whether treatment continuation is required. Where people have struggled for many years with migraines, and have suddenly found an effective treatment (as is gratifyingly frequently the case with the mAbs), there is of course a natural reluctance to take the risk of stopping treatment and the migraines coming back. Some patients will become psychologically dependent on their treatment, and it is important that expectations of what might happen when treatment is stopped are properly managed, so that a sudden worsening does not become a self-fulfilling prophecy, or nocebo effect. It is useful to point out that the half-life of these drugs is around twenty to twenty-five days, and that levels of the mAbs in the system therefore only fall slowly and steadily over time; there is no reason for migraine control to suddenly 'fall off a cliff'. An understanding that a certain proportion of people may be able to successfully stop preventive treatment, and a reassurance that if this is not the case then treatment will be resumed, gives the clinician and the patient the best chance of a positive outcome in this process.

Cluster headache also involves the release of CGRP, and acute attacks may respond to parenteral triptans. Trials of the mAbs have also been undertaken in this condition, with largely disappointing results. One trial of galcanezumab suggested that a single dose of this medication might shorten a cluster headache bout, but the quality of evidence for this effect was not sufficient to allow its adoption for this purpose in the NHS in the UK. A recent observational study from an American centre suggests that monthly injections of galcanezumab may reduce the frequency of attacks over time in patients with chronic cluster headache. Further research is needed in this area.

Overall, the CGRP mAbs are fantastic new additions to our treatment options for headache disorders, particularly migraine. They have very significantly improved the quality of life for many patients who have failed to respond to many other options in the past. They are not panaceas, we need to know more about any long-term adverse effects that might result from their use, and we are still working out how best to use them in the medium to long term, but the world for many migraine sufferers has been made a lot brighter with these treatments, and it is likely that other drugs that target this same pathway will do the same in the future.

How is cluster headache treated?

> *In few conditions are patients so grateful for the relief of their symptoms.*
>
> *British Medical Journal* (1975)[18]

Cluster headache is routinely described as the most severe and debilitating of all primary headache disorders. Proper treatment of cluster headache is often delayed by a lack of correct diagnosis. On average, patients with cluster headache live with the condition for eight years before they get a diagnosis; in part this is due to the episodic nature of the condition in about 80 per cent of patients. Cluster occurs in bouts, typically lasting a few weeks at a time. In a lot of cases, patients will suffer or self-medicate, and by the time they have been through over-the-counter options and found them ineffective, the bout starts to settle, and they do not seek medical attention.

Once a diagnosis has been made, however, there are a number of potentially effective treatment options that should be considered. When people are in a bout, and are having cluster attacks, there are only two types of treatment that have been shown in properly conducted clinical trials to be reliably helpful in taking the pain away: inhaled high concentration oxygen, and non-tablet forms of the triptans. Oxygen inhalation will abort a cluster attack in 70 to 80 per cent of cases, but it must be delivered at a high flow (12–15 litres/minute) and 100 per cent concentration to be properly effective. Oxygen can be prescribed by GPs and specialists in the UK, and is delivered on a regional basis by a small number of companies. In recent years cluster headache has been added to the standard list of conditions for which oxygen prescription is available, and the delivery companies are now for the most part aware of the equipment that is required to allow cluster patients the correct concentration and flow rate. Oxygen cylinders are bulky, of course, and not particularly suitable for use outside the home (although smaller portable cylinders can be obtained with some effort). It is also the case that oxygen cannot be prescribed to patients who smoke because of the obvious dangers of this combination (though there are no reports in the literature of a patient with cluster headache ever blowing themselves up in this way).

The triptans were shown as early as 1991 to be an effective treatment for cluster headache as well as migraine. Because of the generally shorter duration of cluster attacks in comparison with migraine, parenteral administration of the triptans (that is, via a nasal spray or, best of all, via subcutaneous injection) is preferable in cluster headache, and indeed is the only method of administration that has been shown to be effective in clinical trials.

Many cluster patients will have several attacks each day, and this often raises concerns about the amount of triptans that they can get through in a short amount of time. Many GPs are quite properly aware of the possibility of medical overuse, but, as outlined in the section on that condition (see page 71), this seems only to be a genuine problem in people with a personal or strong family history of migraine. Migraine is of course very common, and it is perfectly possible for people to suffer from both cluster headache and migraine, and there are cases where someone with a background propensity to migraine will develop more pervasive headaches as a result of the frequent use of triptans for their cluster attacks. However, under most circumstances, cluster patients do not experience tachyphylaxis (increased frequency of attacks) as a consequence of using triptans more than once a day, and it is good practice to ensure that episodic cluster sufferers are prescribed as many triptans as they need to get them through their bout.

Since the 1970s, doctors have given patients with cluster headache courses of steroids to shorten or abort a bout. This is now known as a transitional treatment. Short courses of steroids will help damp down bouts in perhaps 30 to 50 per cent of cases, and will sometimes abort a bout altogether. Patients should be warned about the potential side effects of steroid use (covered above in the section on medication overuse headache (see page 77)). It is sometimes possible, where people have very short bouts, to use steroids to manage them in their entirety; in other cases they can provide a brief respite (or transition) pending the introduction of other treatments. Greater occipital nerve blocks can also be useful for this purpose in perhaps one-third of cases.

If patients have more prolonged bouts, or have the chronic form of the condition, they may need regular preventive treatment to control their attacks. The preventive treatment of choice for cluster headache is verapamil, a calcium channel-blocking medication originally developed to treat high blood pressure. This seems to be a particularly useful drug for cluster headache, though it is sometimes necessary to build patients up to quite high doses to bring the condition under control (often rather higher than are typically used for blood pressure). Verapamil can cause light-headedness and constipation. If patients go on to this medication, they should have regular ECGs to monitor the electrical activity of the heart, as in a very small number of cases, verapamil can cause heart block – that is, slowing down or even stopping altogether the transmission of electrical signals from the top half of the heart to the bottom half, potentially disrupting normal cardiac function (although most people with more minor forms of heart block do not experience any symptoms from it). Like most preventive treatments, verapamil should be started at a low dose and steadily built up (if tolerated) to a level that brings the attacks under control. If patients are known to have episodic cluster headache, then it should be continued for a few weeks before being brought back down again, in the expectation that the bout will have settled in the meantime. Patients with chronic cluster headache may need longer spells of treatment, but even in these cases the natural history of the disorder means that verapamil is very rarely required in the very long term.

If verapamil is not helpful or tolerated, then there are a number of other options. Currently, many patients will opt for a trial of a handheld non-invasive vagal nerve stimulation (VNS) device as this is available on the NHS in the UK for patients whose condition is not controlled by verapamil. This device is covered in the section on neuromodulation (see page 119).

Traditionally patients with cluster headache might be given lithium. This can still be a very helpful drug for refractory cluster headache, and indeed other refractory headache disorders, but it requires careful monitoring with regular blood tests to ensure blood levels are within safe limits. Lithium toxicity can cause serious neurological and kidney problems. Other preventive medications that can potentially be used for cluster headache include anti-epilepsy drugs such as topiramate, sodium valproate and gabapentin.

Clinical trials have shown that melatonin can sometimes help people with cluster headache. Cluster attacks often wake people in the night; this is thought to be due to involvement of the hypothalamus, which contains the body's own internal body clock, in cluster pathophysiology. The hypothalamus produces melatonin to prepare the brain and body for sleep, and treating people with this medication may impact upon sleep architecture (as mentioned in the section on sleep as a trigger for headaches – see page 122). Melatonin is generally safe and well tolerated, and whilst it is rarely the most effective cluster headache treatment, it is always worth considering for people who have not responded to first-line options.

Patients with refractory chronic cluster headache may ultimately be referred for invasive interventions such as sphenopalatine ganglion or occipital nerve stimulation. There has also been an interest in deep brain stimulation for this condition over the years.

What non-invasive neuromodulation options are available for headaches?

If I apply a magnetic pulse on salt water – that's your brains by the way – it'll generate electric currents, and the electric current in the brain can erase a migraine headache.

Robert Fischell, TED talk, 'My Wish:
Three unusual medical interventions' (2005)[19]

In the five years either side of 2010, there was a lull in the development of new migraine drugs based on CGRP. The excitement of the first generation 'gepants' had fallen away after they were discovered to cause liver problems and had to be withdrawn. It seemed like a significant reappraisal was underway in this area of research. After a series of disappointing trials, a patient population was identified, and a protocol developed for the use of Botox in chronic migraine, but there was a gap into which a series of new treatments emerged, all based on the principle of non-invasive neuromodulation – that is, changing the external peripheral inputs that feed into the central circuits that generate headaches. A number of these treatments have made it into clinical practice and remain available for headache treatment.

Transcranial magnetic stimulation (TMS)

In 2010, a small trial was published in the journal *The Lancet Neurology*, demonstrating the ability of a single pulse of transcranial magnetic stimulation to treat migraine attacks. TMS devices had been used in neurological, and specifically migraine research, for over twenty years. Studies done by Ed Chronicle and his team, initially at Lancaster University and subsequently at the University of Hawaii, had shown that by external magnetic stimulation of the surface of the occipital lobe (the visual part of the brain), one could create the experience of seeing flashes of light (photopsias). They also showed that the threshold at which this would happen was lower in people who had migraines that were triggered by bright lights; in other words, that such people were particularly sensitive to visual stimuli. They demonstrated that this could be reversed by treatment with some of the standard preventive medications that were in use for migraine. It had of course been known for several decades that the processes of migraine aura occurred on the cortical surface, and it was therefore speculated that TMS of the relevant part of the occipital cortex might abort an episode of aura and thereby prevent the subsequent migraine headache from happening.

The results of the trial were broadly positive but the details of what happened were slightly surprising – it seemed to be the case that TMS did not in fact stop the aura process, but it did reduce or prevent the succeeding headache. Single-pulse TMS was eventually approved for use in the UK and Europe, and in 2015 NICE issued a technology assessment that suggested that the treatment could be considered for use in the NHS in England and Wales. It is not widely available on the NHS, as the NICE ruling did not compel funding bodies to provide for it. Individual requests or local systems have to be set up to use it, which are time-consuming and logistically tricky. Nonetheless it can be a useful option in situations where patients cannot tolerate existing acute treatments, or they are contraindicated. Subsequent real-world data suggests that the regular use of TMS can reduce migraine frequency and severity in some cases; more data would be helpful here.

It remains very much an open question as to how TMS works in migraine. Recent research suggests that, rather than stopping aura, stimulation of the cortex alters the exchange of information between the surface of the brain and some of the deeper structures (in particular, the thalamus) that are involved in pain processing, and that it is this that mediates the beneficial effects seen in some patients who use this device.

Vagal nerve stimulation

Back in 2012 I was accosted by a young representative of a medical device company; his name was Paul. Paul had a new machine to show me, about which he was hugely, almost overwhelmingly enthusiastic. This was the first generation of the GammaCore vagal nerve stimulator (VNS). I listened patiently to Paul's pitch, and enquired politely whether the company had acquired any actual evidence that the machine could be helpful for treating migraine. Paul had to admit that at that stage there was no actual evidence as such, but that plans were afoot to run some clinical trials. I said I would be interested to see the results of them. A couple of years later some early studies were published that did indeed show that the VNS device could be helpful both as an acute treatment for migraine and (when used regularly) as a preventive treatment in both migraine and cluster headache. The evidence was always rather more convincing for the latter, and in 2018 the GammaCore VNS device was approved for use on the NHS in the UK as a treatment to prevent or reduce cluster headache in patients who had not responded to the standard first-line preventive therapy, verapamil. In the USA, the device gained FDA approval for use in migraine as well.

The vagus nerve takes information from the brain to the heart, the lungs, the gut and other viscera. More importantly for its potential role in migraine, it takes sensory information back up from those parts of the body to the brain, feeding signals straight into the sensory processing systems that become activated in migraine and cluster headache. Stimulating the vagus nerve seemed to have a positive knock-on effect in turning down these systems, both immediately and more generally over a period of time. VNS, like TMS, is attractive because it is essentially completely safe, and can be used in situations where painkillers are ineffective, or contraindicated, including during pregnancy. Like TMS, clinical experience suggests that a small proportion of patients do very well with this treatment; however, it is not possible to pick out ahead of time who these responders will be.

Supraorbital nerve stimulation

In 2013/14, the Cefaly device, a supraorbital nerve stimulator, was licensed, and reports appeared of patients' early experiences with it. The supraorbital nerve is a branch of the first division of the trigeminal nerve, which has frequently been implicated in migraine pathogenesis over the years. On a very basic level, many patients find that massaging their forehead during an attack will bring some degree of relief. The Cefaly device is similar to the TENS (transdermal electric nerve stimulation) machine used by patients to treat back pain. No properly conducted clinical trials of the Cefaly device have ever been published, but data on real-world experience suggest that it may be helpful for some patients. I have certainly heard plenty of patients tell me that it provides a calming sensation, which can be helpful in getting through their migraines, even if there is little effect on the actual level of pain. It is difficult to shake the feeling, however, that supraorbital nerve stimulators ought to be able to work a little better than this, and other devices are being trialled, including one that stimulates the supraorbital and occipital nerves at the same time, for which preliminary data are encouraging.

Remote electrical stimulation

Think back to when you were a child and were running in the playground, or along a road. When you tripped over and scraped your knee, what did you do (apart from cry, of course)? Chances are you rubbed the affected knee and this, to a greater or lesser extent, distracted you from the pain of the injury. The success of this technique is explained by the longstanding 'gate control theory' of pain, first created by Melzack and Wall in 1965, by which alternative input into pain processing has been shown to interfere with pain signals, and thereby decrease their effect. Using this as a template, an uncomfortable but not painful sensation in the forearm has been shown to decrease migraine intensity and duration. A device based on this finding – the Nerivon – has been licensed for use in the USA.

What lifestyle modifications can help reduce headaches?

Headache likes people to be a bit boring. It likes people to eat regularly, to sleep regularly, to keep well hydrated and not overdo things. In other words, to live a moderate life. Of course, it is not always possible to live such a life all the time, nor is it desirable. Over the years I have met people who have been so assiduous in avoiding any situation that might bring on a headache, that they have ended up living very narrow, contained lives, largely free of headaches, but also free of the joys of spontaneity. However, there are things that one can do to try to reduce the impact of irregularities of lifestyle on an underlying tendency to headaches, and particularly migraines. The fact that many of these interventions, or changes in the pattern of living, are generally good for one's well-being and productivity is a bonus.

The three most important areas for attention are sleep, what we eat and drink, and how we arrange our working day.

Sleep

'O sleep! O gentle sleep! Nature's soft nurse.'
William Shakespeare, *Henry IV, Part II*[20]

The relationship between headaches and sleep is complex, but in general people are more likely to get headaches, particularly migraines, if their normal sleep pattern is disturbed. Usually this means sleep deprivation due to insomnia of some sort, but occasionally it can mean sleeping in too late, which will set off migraines in some patients. Those who wake up early in the mornings tend, on average, to have their attacks earlier in the day; night owls, on the other hand, tend to have attacks later on. There are various things that can go wrong with sleep. One can have difficulty with sleep initiation (getting off to sleep in the first place), one can experience sleep fragmentation (waking up frequently at night and struggling to get back to sleep), or one can have what appears to be sufficient quantities of undisturbed sleep, but nonetheless wake unrefreshed. At its worst, insomnia can lead to excessive tiredness in the day. If you experience a significant tendency to fall asleep during the day, for example when sitting quietly after a meal, or as a passenger (or worse still, a driver) in a car sitting in a queue of traffic, or when watching television or a film, then you should have your sleep properly assessed, as you may have an underlying problem such as sleep apnea.

For many headache sufferers, daytime somnolence is not so much of an issue, but poor sleep is nonetheless important in triggering or exacerbating their tendency to headaches. One initial approach to this is to follow what are called sleep hygiene recommendations. The fundamental point of these is to reinforce the normal compartmentalisation of the 24-hour day into sleep and wake cycles. The brain should naturally prepare for sleep by various physiological changes, most importantly the release of the hormone melatonin from the hypothalamus. The brain releases melatonin at intervals during the day, but there should be a large burst in the mid evening to prepare us for a good night's sleep. (Release of melatonin around lunchtime contributes to the common feeling of mild sleepiness that hits many of us in the mid afternoon.) These natural physiological processes can be reinforced by routine; such a routine can also reduce the possibility of interference in sleep initiation by factors such as excess caffeine intake, and lower the chance of sleep fragmentation caused, for example, by having to get up in the night to urinate.

It can be helpful, therefore, not to eat an evening meal too late. Caffeinated drinks should be avoided past mid afternoon, and one should not drink too much fluid in the evening, to reduce the need to get up in the night to empty one's bladder. It is useful to develop a wind-down routine. A bath or shower can be helpful as part of this. Set aside ten to fifteen minutes to think about what you have been doing that day, and prepare for what is coming tomorrow. This can reduce (though probably not completely remove) the tendency to lie awake worrying about work, family issues or other things. You should set a reasonable time for going to bed and, most importantly, for getting up in the morning, and stick to it, trying not to vary the latter by more than an hour, even at weekends or on holiday. Avoid napping in the day if at all possible. Recent research recommends getting up at the same time every day is perhaps the most important thing that one can do, to consolidate good sleep habits. The bedroom should be kept cool, dark and quiet. It is for sleep and sexual intercourse only. You should make sure that you do not use a smartphone, tablet or laptop within an hour of going to sleep; the light from these devices interferes with the brain's production of melatonin. You should not watch television or listen to the radio in the bedroom. If you live in a small flat or a bedsit, you should try as much as possible to separate where you live and work in the daytime from where you go to bed at night. Avoid sitting or lying on the bed to work during the day, for example.

Pharmaceutical aids to sleep can be helpful, particularly if the problem is initiating sleep, but the effect of these wears off pretty quickly, and as a general rule it is inadvisable to take sleeping tablets for more than seven to ten days in a row. If you have a very abnormal sleep phase (most usually this means that you are a night owl, whose brain doesn't want to turn off until the small hours of the morning), taking melatonin in bursts of two weeks at a time (perhaps two or three times in a row, with a week's break in between) can be a useful way to start to reset that sleep phase, in much the same way that people use melatonin to treat jet lag. Advanced sleep phase

– that is, a tendency to go to sleep in the early evening, and then be awake again by 2–3 a.m. – is much rarer; people with this condition seem more likely to also experience migraines.

The underlying sleep pattern of most people with headaches is basically normal, but sleep can be easily disrupted by the normal intrusions of daily life (often anxiety about work, family and so on), and then once normal sleep patterns are lost, they can be very difficult to recover. Vicious cycles can emerge in which poor sleep causes more headaches, which in turn interferes with sleep, which then causes more headaches, and so on. Sleep hygiene is an important way of trying to make sleep patterns more regular, and more normal. It is something, to a greater or lesser extent, which most people with recurrent or chronic headaches will find it helpful to address.

If sleep hygiene does not do the trick, then there is very good evidence that cognitive behavioural therapy specifically directed at improving sleep quality (known as CBT-I) can help. For patients with migraine, sleep compression has been shown to work better than sleep restriction, particularly for people with a chronic form of the condition. Indeed, one trial published fifteen years ago demonstrated that this form of intervention on its own could help patients revert from a chronic form of migraine to an episodic form. There are now digital methods of delivering this treatment. Details are given in the resources section at the end of this book (see page 171).

Food and drink

> *I had this terrific headache all of a sudden. I wished to God*
> *old Mrs Antolini would come in with the coffee.*
> J.D. Salinger, *The Catcher in the Rye* (1951)[21]

Contrary to widespread and repeated claims, there is no such thing as a headache or migraine diet. No properly conducted clinical trial has ever shown that following one type of diet over another can reliably and reproducibly reduce the tendency to headaches or migraines. However, large-scale studies of migraine triggers show that missing meals, and certain foodstuffs, are important migraine triggers. Like all questions of trigger management and lifestyle modification, it is important to remember that these are not triggers for everybody. If your headaches are not routinely triggered by cheese, chocolate or alcohol, that does not mean that they are not migraines. Similarly, if your headaches are not triggered by any of the aforementioned foodstuffs, then there is no real point in cutting them completely out of your diet, as it is unlikely to improve matters.

The commonest food- and drink-related migraine triggers are missing meals, and dehydration. It is of course possible to avoid both of these with fairly simple planning. With regard to fluid intake, there is no particular maximum or minimum, but most authorities would recommend that people drink at least 2–3 litres of fluid each day. Caffeine, as mentioned in the section on acute treatment of headaches (see page 66), can be a useful adjunct to standard painkillers, but exposure to too much caffeine, too regularly, can start to make people feel more headachy. It is therefore sensible to restrict caffeine intake to no more than a couple of caffeinated drinks per day. It is useful to be aware that a lot of artificial soft drinks do contain a lot of caffeine, as well as the more obvious tea and coffee. Some forms of tea and coffee are naturally caffeine-free, but you should check carefully, as this will not necessarily be the case. Decaffeinated drinks do contain small amounts of caffeine, but usually no more than 10–15 per cent of the amount contained in the equivalent quantity of the normally caffeinated variety.

Alcohol is quite a frequent trigger for headaches of various types. Perhaps 20 per cent of patients with migraine will find that alcohol brings on an attack, not typically immediately, but usually after a few hours. (This fact was used back in the 1980s by researchers who wanted to trigger migraines reliably at a set time so that they could study them; the use of alcohol to do this would not get past twenty-first-century research ethics committees . . .) For most patients with migraine, alcohol triggering manifests predominantly as a tendency to much more severe hangovers than might be expected for the amount of alcohol consumed. Patients with cluster headache may find that alcohol will trigger an attack almost instantly if they are in a bout, but not at all at other times. Some people find that the effect of alcohol varies according to what exactly has been consumed. Again, there is very little consistency to this. Some people tolerate wine but not beer, or vice versa. Others find that red wine triggers headaches, but white wine does not. Yet others find themselves particularly sensitive to champagne or other sparkling wines. As always with headaches, it is best to practise moderation, and even if alcohol does not appear to be a particularly important trigger, to keep well within the national recommended limits for adult men and women.

With regard to food, many people worry that particular items, such as cheese or chocolate will bring on headaches. However, it is far more likely that missing meals brings on attacks. I used to share an office with an otherwise very astute neurologist who at regular intervals would return to the office at lunchtime in the throes of a migraine, knowing full well that it was because she had skipped breakfast and had had nothing to eat during the morning.

Exactly why this is, is not fully understood. It does not seem to be directly related to blood sugar levels. The best advice is to eat sensibly and well, with a balanced diet, and to ensure that meals are not missed. Some people are sensitive to well-known triggers such as cheese or chocolate, as well as to other substances such as monosodium glutamate (MSG – a flavouring used in Chinese and other oriental foods); migraine sufferers may notice that other specific foods may set off attacks – citrus fruit or onion and garlic are mentioned not infrequently. There has been a drive to dismiss these reports over recent years as being manifestations of the types of food-craving that can be experienced as a premonitory or prodromal symptom in migraine, but many patients do not experience any form of craving, but simply and reliably report a tendency of migraine to come on some time after exposure to particular substances.

Most people who live with headaches over any length of time come to realise what foodstuffs are a problem for them, and if they can (and want to), they will generally avoid them. It is in my experience very rarely the case that there is an unexpected intolerance that underlies a tendency to headaches, and undergoing an extensive exclusion diet is very unlikely to be informative or revealing. There remains no convincing evidence that migraine or other headaches relate in any widespread manner to any form of food allergy. Studies done using commercially available allergy tests suggest that cutting out foods to which the tests are positive generally makes very little difference to migraine frequency.

The question is often asked whether migraine and headaches are a feature of coeliac disease, or more generally of gluten or lactose intolerance. Again, over the years I have seen a few patients in whom cutting out wheat or dairy products has been a helpful thing to do, but with the benefit of hindsight it has been the case that these patients almost all had other symptoms (abdominal pain, bloating or abnormal stools) that hinted at the presence of this problem, rather than presenting with just headaches alone. Again, there is no indication that patients with headache should try excluding these substances from their diet, or have blood tests for coeliac disease.

Over the last decade, there has been increasing interest in the role that the gut, and in particular the bacteria that are found within it – the microbiome – might play in the development of neurological disorders. Very intriguing data is starting to emerge, for example, linking the presence of certain bacteria in the gut with the chances of developing Parkinson's disease. For headache disorders, the question has been asked whether consuming probiotics – that is, specific cultures of certain bacteria – might help reduce migraines, in particular. A couple of early studies suggest that this might be possible, to a degree at least. It is too early to routinely recommend probiotics to people with headache disorders, but this is an area about which knowledge is likely to develop rapidly in the next decade.

Work

Headaches were like birds. Starlings. They could be perfectly calm, then a single acorn could drop and send the entire flock to the sky.

Erika Swyler, *The Mermaid Girl: A Story* (2016)[22]

Most adults spend the vast majority of the day at work, going to work, or coming home from work. Work provides a major source of life satisfaction, but also of anxiety, of physical and mental stress. It is unsurprising, therefore, that issues around work may play important parts in triggering or exacerbating a tendency to headaches or migraines.

Some of the problems that can arise from work have already been alluded to in previous sections. Work anxiety can cause sleep difficulties. Work patterns, especially shift work, can be highly disruptive to sleep patterns, and can be problematic for people with a propensity to headaches. In some cases, shift working is simply not viable for people with headaches, and this fact should be borne in mind when looking for jobs, as well as when one is employed in a job that uses shift-working patterns. Similarly, the demands of work scheduling may make it difficult for people with headaches to keep hydrated or eat regular meals. For the most part these are not intentional problems (they certainly shouldn't be), but simply arise over time because of ever-increasing demands on the sufferer's time.

Many people are largely sedentary during the working day, and increasingly we all spend an ever-greater proportion of our time sitting in front of a computer screen. This can put strain on the neck, in particular, especially if the screen and keyboard are not optimally positioned. Large companies will have – or employ – occupational health teams who should carry out ergonomic assessments of the workplace for people with medical problems, including headache disorders. Smaller companies should be aware of these issues, and prepared to make the relatively small changes that will be helpful for their employees who are prone to headaches.

It is important to have regular breaks in the working day. Such breaks allow people to eat and drink, and go to the toilet, but also to stretch and mobilise, thereby reducing the adverse consequences of prolonged immobility. Again, a particular problem of modern working life is the effect of relative immobility on the neck. Neck tightness and stiffness may build up over the course of a long working day in front of a computer screen, leading to abnormal sensory signals feeding straight into the bit of the brain (the trigeminocervical complex) that generates many headache disorders, including migraine and cluster headache. This has the potential to set up a vicious cycle in which neck strain starts to cause more headaches, which then generate more neck stiffness and discomfort, which in turn cause more headaches, and so on.

Employers do have a responsibility to their employees under disability legislation. Headache disorders, including migraine, are not necessarily classified as disabilities, but they may be if they cause symptoms that are sufficiently debilitating, sufficiently common, and have been going on sufficiently long to meet the criteria set out in the Disability Act. It should not really be necessary for someone's headaches to meet these formal criteria to precipitate a review of workspace and working practices, but certainly if a person has a chronic, debilitating headache disorder, then 'reasonable adjustments' should be made to their workspace and work schedules to prevent work-related issues making their medical condition worse, insofar as it is possible to do so.

For patients with chronic migraine, for example, this might include looking at the effect of ambient lighting and computer screen brightness settings, so as to reduce the impact of light inputs on a tendency to photophobia. It might include moving a migraine sufferer into a quieter area of the office to prevent the adverse effect of excessive noise, or altering hours of work to accommodate sleep disturbances or to reduce the impact of a stressful commute. There may be a discussion about working from home, or following some form of hybrid working practice, to improve the patient's control over their work environment, and thereby their productivity.

There is extremely good evidence that chronic migraine, in particular, is associated with high levels of absenteeism. Equally problematic, if not more so, is presenteeism – that is, when people go into work when they should not do so because of illness. Lack of understanding of headache disorders, and prejudice against people who suffer from them, may lead to such sufferers being reluctant to call in sick, because they fear that the reality of their medical problem may be doubted, and that this will ultimately lead to problems, up to and including disciplinary measures and dismissal. In my experience, migraine is not infrequently used as an excuse or pretext by poor managers (often outright bullies) to laud it over those underneath them, and to exert power over them. This of course only exacerbates the underlying tendency to headaches or migraines, and itself can make the situation worse, often resulting in a crisis when people are off sick for a long time, sometimes never returning at all.

Conversely, a cooperative and sympathetic approach to managing the workspace and working practices of people with headache disorders brings benefits not only to the sufferers themselves, but also to their companies, in terms of improved productivity. Migraine is estimated to cost the UK economy billions of pounds each year. Some of that is inevitable, but much of that lost GDP could be reduced by improved diagnosis, better treatment and more positive attitudes to people with headache disorders within the world of work.

What alternative treatments are known to help headaches?

Prescription and over-the-counter medications play an important role for many people coping with chronic pain. The bottom line is that effective pain management can include many different approaches that include pain medications with complementary therapies such as yoga and massage. There is no one-size-fits-all solution.

Naomi Judd, interview with
The Caregiver's Voice (2011)[23]

Prior to the nineteenth century, there were no alternative therapies – there were just therapies. It wasn't until the middle of that century that the boundaries of what counted as scientific medicine, and indeed of science itself, were established in universities, laboratories, hospitals, journals and learned societies. This process of professionalisation designated certain ways of doing medicine as approved, orthodox and 'scientific', and others as alternative, pseudoscientific and quackery. Mesmerism, for example, started out as a scientific endeavour, achieving significant benefits in pain control and anaesthesia, before being overtaken by ether and then chloroform. Not only did mesmerism become outmoded, it became branded as unorthodox, and its practitioners were for the most part actively excluded from the mid-century medical profession.

When it comes to headache treatments, there are certainly no shortage of alternative approaches. Two minutes on any internet search engine will demonstrate this. Many practitioners of alternative therapies will not recognise the validity of scientific methods of testing their treatments, such as randomised clinical trials, but there is such evidence to back at least one alternative therapy – perhaps the oldest one still in regular use – and that one is acupuncture.

Headache is mentioned in some of the oldest extant works of Chinese medicine (such as *The Yellow Emperor's Classic of Internal Medicine*, which is thought to date from the second millennium BCE), and acupuncture has been used as a treatment option from those earliest days. A trial performed in Germany two decades ago demonstrated that patients with chronic migraine who were given acupuncture experienced fewer headaches than an equivalent population who had been given a sham procedure. Interestingly, however, a third set of patients who had acupuncture needles inserted at random points in the scalp (as opposed to traditional acupuncture points along the lines of Qi) also did better than those who had the sham procedure. The implication of this is that sticking needles into people's heads may make them less headachy, and that it doesn't matter too much where you put them. Certainly the high placebo rates seen in the trials of Botox for migraine might support this interpretation.

On the basis of this and other trials, acupuncture has been recommended as a treatment option in the NHS, but it is very difficult to find practitioners of this type of treatment within the NHS these days. Many patients do find acupuncture helpful, and the recommendation that one should have up to ten sessions is probably sensible, as fewer than that number may not be sufficient to get a proper sense of whether it is helping.

This is pretty much where the evidence base for alternative therapies starts and ends. As will be clear from the sections on lifestyle modifications and on the role of the neck in headache, physical therapies directed at keeping the neck supple and as pain-free as possible certainly can be beneficial for many patients with headaches, though no trials have ever been undertaken to compare the various different forms of physical therapy (osteopathy, chiropractic and so on) against one another in this patient population.

Beyond this, we are very much in an evidence-free zone. Many patients find interactions with alternative practitioners helpful. This of course may be due to a harnessing of the expectation effect – that is, the tendency of medical conditions to improve when people expect that they will do so. In scientific medicine, the expectation effect, when it is positive, is known as the placebo effect; when negative, it is called the nocebo effect. This can occur when, from previous experience, people do not believe their treatment will work; in the trials of the new CGRP monoclonal antibodies, for example, the placebo effect in patients who had previously failed two or three other treatments (an average improvement of about one day per month, despite not being given active medication), disappeared in those who had previously failed four treatments, to be replaced by a nocebo effect of a worsening of one to two days per month (though the positive effect of the antibody itself was preserved). The take home message is that, for alternative therapies as much as for standard therapies, the power of a positive and constructive interaction with the practitioner cannot be over-estimated.

There are few alternative therapies that I actively discourage patients from trying. I personally do not see the point of homeopathy, but rationales can be made for the potential benefit of most physical therapies. I am agnostic about the effect of daith piercing (a procedure in which a pin is put through the area just anterior to the external auditory canal, an area that (uniquely) is innervated by the vagus nerve); whilst very few of my patients have found it helpful in any way, I acknowledge that there might be a selection bias in action (i.e. that there may be plenty of satisfied daith-pierced headache-free people walking around who do not need to come to see me), but without further published data on the long-term outcomes of this intervention, it is difficult to say.

I do suggest that people are very wary of any surgical approach to managing headaches. Many such interventions have been touted over the years as the ultimate solution to the problem of living with headaches. Time and data have not been kind to any of them. The most recent iteration of this is corrugator surgery, in which the corrugator muscles (which are the ones that allow us to frown) are removed. The idea behind this is that these muscles are compressing the supraorbital nerves that run through them, and that this is in turn driving people's migraines. This is not the most ridiculous of concepts, but experience (and brain anatomy and physiology) suggests that it is very unlikely that this is the sole driving factor behind most people's migraines. The published data on this intervention is of questionable quality, and anecdotally many people who undergo it have a brief honeymoon period during which their headaches improve, before everything goes back to baseline.

It is wise to be constructively agnostic about alternative therapies. So long as the proposed intervention is safe, and the proposed duration of treatment is sensible (no miracle cures, and no indefinite courses), and one can approach things with an open but positive mindset, alternative therapies may have a part to play in helping people live with their headaches. Some may even in time cross the boundary and become part of the headache orthodoxy.

Frequently asked questions

What can I expect out of a headache consultation?

> *If migraine patients have a common and legitimate second complaint besides their migraines, it is that they have not been listened to by physicians. Looked at, investigated, drugged, charged, but not listened to.*
>
> Oliver Sacks, *Migraine* (1970)[24]

To paraphrase the American satirist Tom Lehrer, a consultation with a headache specialist is like a sewer: what you get out of it depends on what you put in to it. Setting aside scatological allusions, the point is that the more information you bring with you to a consultation, the better. If you have read through some of the chapters of this book, you will understand the sort of things that a headache specialist might be interested in; for example, when your headaches started, how frequently they occur, what they feel like, how they effect your daily life, and so on. It is useful to keep a diary for a period prior to a consultation (and remember to bring it with you); a paper record is fine, or a printout from an app-based diary. Of particular importance, especially if the purpose of the consultation is to talk about new treatment, is to try to put together a list of those treatments you have been given in the past. Be as specific as you can be; any information about what medicines you have taken, at what dose and for how long, how helpful (or not) it was, and whether it caused any side effects, is useful. Don't just say, 'I've tried everything!' – even if it feels like you have, you won't have done. This information may be vital if you are being considered for advanced treatments on the NHS, as funding may depend on your headache specialist being able to show that you have tried a number of previous options.

If you have had previous investigations, such as blood tests or scans, then bring copies of results if you can. Details of any other medical problems, and any medication prescribed for them, are important.

There is then the vexed question of whether, if you have done your own research about your headaches and have questions or theories relating to this, you should present your specialist with a file of printouts from websites or academic papers. I personally am always happy to look through anything that someone has taken the time to put together, though it may not always be possible to do it there and then.

Having brought all this information to the table, what might you then expect your specialist to do? After going through the history of your headaches, and any other related medical or social information, and examining you (if appropriate), you can first and foremost expect a diagnosis. This is the first step, from which everything else can follow. There is little excuse for a clinician not to give you at least a working diagnosis (or diagnoses), as unclassifiable headaches are really very rare. Ideally you will then be given options for acute treatment and, if necessary, options for medications or other interventions that prevent, reduce or ameliorate your headaches. In some cases it may be appropriate for you to have a rescue or emergency plan, for medications that can be used at home, or in an emergency department, if your headaches run out of control.

If appropriate, you may be referred for investigations, such as blood tests or scans. Finally, you have some form of agreement about whether you need a follow-up review, and if so, when (roughly) it will be and what information you will collect in the meantime and bring back for review so that the success (or otherwise) of your treatment plan can be assessed.

Don't worry if you don't have all of this information (very few people do), but the more you can bring to the table, the more you are likely to get out of your consultation. Similarly, you should not be concerned if not all your questions are answered at your first visit, so long as further reviews are planned, if necessary.

Finally, it is common in the twenty-first-century NHS for those who are seen by headache specialists not to be routinely offered follow-up appointments, because of the scarcity of headache resources within the service. In these circumstances, you may be discharged with a series of options for treatment for you and your general practitioner to work through. Given the demands on the time of most GPs, it is important not to assume that they will read through the headache specialist's letters in detail, and contact you proactively to initiate or change treatment. The onus will be on you to drive this process; you may need to be politely persistent in getting your prescriptions written or changed.

Do I need a brain scan?

> *'On your thirtieth birthday, you said you couldn't see. On your thirty-fourth birthday, you forgot my name for an hour. Last year, when I asked you what you wanted, you said a CAT scan.'*
>
> *'I had a headache.'*
>
> From the script for *City Slickers* (1991)[25]

One of the most common questions I am asked by patients who consult me with headache is whether they need a brain scan. Before answering this question it's worth considering why people should think that having a scan would be useful in the first instance. In part this is due to the enormously pervasive cultural link between headaches and serious brain pathology such as tumours or aneurysms. This is a common trope in films, voiced by Woody Allen in *Annie Hall*, Billy Crystal in *City Slickers* and even one of Arnold Schwarzenegger's young pupils in *Kindergarten Cop*. While tumours and aneurysms are fortunately very rare, it is not that uncommon for people to know someone who knows someone whose brother, or cousin, or friend, had headaches and was then diagnosed with a serious brain problem. No one ever asks whether the two facts are connected. Correlation does not always indicate causation, particularly as headaches are so common.

Before the introduction of CT scanning in the 1970s and MRI scanning in the 1980s, it was virtually impossible to see what was going on in the brain *in vivo*. Techniques such as pneumoencephalography (injecting air into the spinal fluid so that it would allow the outline of the brain to be seen on a subsequent plain X-ray) were difficult, painful and gave generally unreliable results that were difficult to interpret. In most cases, a definite diagnosis of a brain tumour was only made during an operation or, more commonly, at a post-mortem.

Nowadays, of course, modern imaging technology makes it relatively straightforward to obtain pictures of the brain. CT and MRI scanning are almost universally available in advanced societies, although they remain an expensive resource within the constraints of a national healthcare system, and their use needs to be carefully controlled, for a number of reasons. CT scans use X-rays, and one should always be mindful of avoiding unnecessary exposure to ionising radiation. CT is very good for looking at bones (e.g. the skull after a head injury, or looking for fractures) and for taking a quick look for things that shouldn't be there, such as blood, a large tumour or an extensive stroke. CT scans can miss more subtle brain pathology, for which MRI scanning is more appropriate. MRI scans take longer, they are more expensive and a scarcer resource than CT.

In addition to these logistical and financial issues, there are clinical limitations to the specificity of imaging. At least 2 per cent of the population have got 'odd brains'. By this I mean that scans often throw up incidental findings that are rarely of any actual significance, but may cause anxiety, could be misinterpreted and may encourage further over-investigation. Examples of such findings include minor brain asymmetries, arachnoid cysts, developmental venous anomalies, calcification of the falx or hyperostosis interna frontalis, or age-related changes in the white matter (the deep parts of the brain largely comprising the axons – the wiring that connects the various parts of the brain together, and the brain with the rest of the body). Sometimes imaging will uncover genuine pathology, such as a meningioma (a benign growth of the lining of the brain) that has nothing to do with the problem for which the scan was done (headache), and which might have caused no particular problems had they remained undiscovered.

One must balance, therefore, the positive aspects of imaging, that is, the finding of genuinely relevant pathology if it is there, versus the downsides, both in terms of engendering anxiety and over-investigation of an individual patient, and the cost to society as a whole of over-investigation. Scans are often requested to allay patient anxiety about an underlying tumour or aneurysm, but good evidence exists to show that the anxiolytic effect of a normal scan is relatively short-lived, usually no longer than six to twelve months, if the patient is not then provided with a proper diagnosis and effective treatment instituted.

My personal practice is never to refuse to scan someone who is worried about their headaches, particularly if they have never had a scan before (I'm generally reluctant to scan someone who has been scanned before 'just in case something has been missed'). However I always counsel people about the risks of an incidental finding so that they are prepared for this if (as in a lot of cases) one shows up.

Under what circumstances, therefore, might a scan be indicated? One would certainly want to take a look in cases of sudden onset, severe (thunderclap) headaches, to make sure that there has been no bleeding or any other sudden change in brain structure to account for this. One would want to arrange scans for patients with headache who have fixed signs on clinical examination, to understand whether there is a structural problem in the brain to account for them. One might arrange imaging for patients with persistent progressive headaches, again to ensure that this is not due to the steady growth of a tumour, or blood-clotting causing raised intracranial pressure. Episodic headaches, that come and go, are very unlikely to be due to any serious brain problem, though they can, and do, have significant impacts upon people's quality of life.

Work done by David Kernick and colleagues about twenty years ago, using the UK national general practice database, clearly shows that if one can diagnose a primary headache disorder such as tension-type headache or migraine (and one should remember that these are by far the commonest causes of headaches in the general population), the probability of that patient having an abnormal brain scan is 0.045 per cent. The bottom line is that while there are no absolute rules for when a scan should be done, most people with headaches do not need scans, and scans should only ever be requested after a proper consideration of the patient's history and examination findings, and what their underlying diagnosis is likely to be from a clinical point of view.

Dr Mark Weatherall

Are headaches hereditary?

In headaches and in worry
Vaguely life leaks away
And Time will have his fancy
To-morrow or to-day.
    W. H. Auden, 'As I Walked Out One Evening' (1940)[26]

It's long been known, at least since the nineteenth century, that some types of headache seem to run in families. In works on migraine written by nineteenth-century neurological luminaries such as Edward Liveing and William Gowers, this was stated clearly. The first report of a family in whom recurrent attacks of what we would now think of as hemiplegic migraine (that is, migraines associated with an aura causing weakness down one side of the body, rather like a stroke) was published in the *British Medical Journal* in 1912. Studies of the relative contributions of the environment and genetics to the development of migraine were published in the mid-twentieth century, but it was not until 1996 that the first specific gene associated with a particular form of migraine was discovered. This was isolated in a Dutch family with a tendency to hemiplegic migraine. The gene was found to code for a protein (CACNA1A) involved in the transport of calcium across cell membranes in the body. It was hypothesised that abnormal function of this channel membrane predisposed to instability within cells on the surface of the brain, which in turn predisposed to the development of more severe forms of migraine aura. Interestingly, different mutations in this gene were found to cause other neurological problems, such as epilepsy or episodic unsteadiness (ataxia). Over the next five years two more genes were isolated in other families with hemiplegic migraines. These were also membrane channel genes, in these cases coding for proteins dealing with the movement of sodium and potassium in and out of cells; changes in all of these proteins affected the release or uptake of glutamate, one of the central neurotransmitters in normal brain function.

However, none of these genetic changes are routinely found in people with standard migraines, whether or not they have aura, or other headache types. Instead, it seems increasingly likely that the predisposition to migraine results from possessing multiple mutations in different genes. The process of trying to sort out multi-genetic conditions like migraine is undertaken by scientists working in genomic medicine, research that aims to link the presence of certain individual clinical features of the condition (such as throbbing pain, nausea, or light and noise sensitivity) with changes in particular areas of the human genome, and thereby to home in on the specific genes that might be responsible. A recent publication in the journal *Nature Genetics* lists over 120 candidate migraine genes. It is interesting to note that these genes are involved in a variety of mechanisms, including the development of blood vessels, the production of neurotransmitters, membrane channels, the laying down of connective tissues, and so on.

What people inherit is the propensity to a particular type of headache. Migraine almost always runs in families, but there are some people who are unfortunate enough to be the only member of the family with the particular combination of, and sufficient numbers of, the relevant genetic changes. Disorders such as cluster headache also have a genetic component to them, though it is much less common for them to run in families.

When taking a family history of migraine at a consultation, I often jokingly say that the patient in front of me knows who to blame for their migraine genes. Sometimes this raises a chuckle, particularly if the aforesaid responsible parent is in the consultation room with the patient, but sometimes it raises no more than a rueful smile, acknowledging that the cards (the genetic cards, in this case) have been stacked against them from the start. It is important to note, however, that whilst one cannot do anything about one's genetic inheritance and one's predilection to headaches, the way that this predisposition plays itself out in people's lives can be very different in each case, and there are many internal and external factors that play into the ultimate outcome of that predisposition.

Likewise, parents should not feel guilty about passing migraine genes on to their children. Firstly, there is nothing you can do about it anyway. Secondly, their migraines (if they get them) are unlikely to be the same as yours. Thirdly, they will benefit from another twenty to thirty years of science applied to the treatment of their condition. And fourthly, perhaps there is (or at least in the past has been) some benefit to having those migraine genes. Otherwise, from an evolutionary point of view, how to explain why so many people have a tendency to transient episodes of neurological dysfunction, and headaches that make us want to hide away in a cool, dark place?

Are headaches different in children?

Little children, headache; big children, heartache.

Italian proverb

Headache disorders are lifelong afflictions. They affect children every bit as much as adults. It's doubly important to recognise severe headache problems in children, and do the best to treat them, because time lost in the formative years of school and socialisation is time that, in some cases, can never be got back. Children are prone to pretty much all the primary and secondary headache problems mentioned in this book, but they may present somewhat differently in children, and it is helpful to recognise this. Migraines, in particular, often manifest themselves very differently in the young. Children are much more likely to have shorter headaches, and to find that a short period of rest or sleep will abolish them altogether. There are particular childhood migraine variants that in some cases do not seem to persist into adulthood. Examples include benign torticollis of childhood, which is almost never seen in adults, and abdominal migraines, which can sometimes persist into adulthood, or even present for the first time at that stage of life (this can cause some diagnostic difficulties). In many cases the childhood variants will settle, but children will then start to experience more typical adult headache symptoms as they enter their teens or early twenties.

Other headache disorders such as cluster headache are fortunately rare in childhood, but they can occur, and it is very important to be aware of this possibility, to allow timely diagnosis and appropriate treatment to be instituted.

When taking a headache history from a child, it is important (as in all paediatric practice) to listen very carefully to what the child has to say, as well as getting a collateral history of the parents or carers, including a description of how the child behaves during attacks. Getting children to draw pictures of their attacks is often a good way to engage with them, and can be illuminating. When children become adolescents, this can be a difficult period, as they may not wish to engage with authority figures such as medical professionals, or do what their parents are telling them to do. It is important to try to encourage increasing independence and self-reliance in managing headache disorders at this stage of life.

Most standard acute treatment options are available for use in children. Childhood doses of paracetamol and non-steroidal anti-inflammatories can be used from the earliest years, and some of the triptans are licensed for use in adolescents. The placebo rates for response to acute medication are very high in childhood, which is of course helpful in clinical practice. Many of the preventive treatments used in adults can also be used in children, if necessary. Careful attention needs to be paid to dosing, and there are options that should not be used, particularly drugs that might have implications for contraception or reproductive health, such as sodium valproate or topiramate. There is an increasing acknowledgement that good-quality preventive options are required for children and adolescents, to prevent the adverse consequences of severe headache disorders on social development and schooling. New options such as the CGRP monoclonal antibodies are being actively studied in these age groups, and should become available for use in due course.

The lifestyle adjustments outlined in earlier sections also apply to children and adolescents, in some cases doubly so.

It is common, for example, for teenagers to develop a delayed sleep phase (that is, to become night owls, whose brains don't want to switch off for sleep until the middle of the night); when, therefore, they are faced with the necessity to get up early in the morning to go to school, this may lead to cumulative sleep deprivation, and increasingly frequent headaches in those who are prone to them. Some countries recognise the deleterious effect of delayed sleep phase in teenagers by introducing a delayed start to the school day in that age group, but if that is not possible, then consideration should be given to sleep hygiene and pharmacological methods to bring sleep onset forward, as outlined in the 'Treatments' chapter (see page 65). Teenagers may be particularly prone to irregularities in routine. Caffeine intake may be unexpectedly high due to consumption of soft drinks aimed at this age group. Whilst teenagers may have very little control over their work (school) day, it is at least the case that, for the most part, the school day is naturally broken up into segments, with breaks in between. Where sixth-formers have some control over their time, those with headaches should be encouraged to follow advice about working in an ergonomically sensible workspace, and build in regular breaks in their schoolwork and revision. As before, these interventions should also make them generally more productive when they work.

Children with headaches, and parents of children with headaches, should be aware that this is often a stage of life when people are headachy, but it is by no means inevitable that this will continue to be the case into adulthood. The author, for one, was plagued with recurrent migraines for most of his teenage years, before they largely settled down in his twenties, appearing thereafter now and again just to remind him that he is, and remains, someone with a propensity to migraines. Whilst this is not the pattern for everyone, by any means, it is not uncommon for the physical, psychological and social stresses of adolescence to feed into a tendency to migraines, and for those processes to play themselves out as people enter adult life.

Are people with headaches at risk of heart disease or stroke?

'I don't want to die now!' he yelled. 'I've still got a head-ache! I don't want to go to heaven with a headache, I'd be all cross and wouldn't enjoy it!'

Douglas Adams, *The Hitchhiker's Guide to the Galaxy* (1979)[27]

Headaches are common. Heart disease and cerebrovascular disease (such as stroke) are also common. Over the course of a lifetime, therefore, many people who suffer from migraine or other headache types will have heart attacks or strokes. Does the fact that they are headache sufferers make it more likely that this will happen?

The answer to this question for the most common of all headaches – tension-type headache – is almost certainly 'no'. There is also no convincing evidence that people who suffer from cluster headache and other rare primary headache disorders are at any greater risk either. For migraine, however, the picture is more complicated, and has evolved as a result of a number of increasingly sophisticated and well-planned epidemiological studies that have appeared over the course of the last twenty-five years.

The bottom line is that suffering from any form of migraine probably does increase your risk of heart disease, but only by a very small amount. It is not a risk that you can do anything about (no studies have ever shown that reducing the frequency of migraines impacts upon risk levels in heart disease or stroke), and in this regard it is the same as the risk brought on by age, or a positive family history. The overall level of risk attributable to migraine is much lower than that associated with any other non-modifiable risk factor.

Similarly, migraine with aura has been shown to be a risk factor for stroke in women between the ages of twenty-one and forty-five. It is for this reason that the use of an oestrogen-containing contraceptive pill (which also increases the risk of stroke at this age) is relatively contraindicated in women who have had migraine with aura. The same has not been shown for migraine without aura, and there is really no convincing evidence that there is any significant increase in male migraine sufferers, or in women over the age of forty-five who have this condition. Common modifiable risk factors – smoking, high blood pressure, diabetes and high cholesterol levels – are much more important than whether you suffer from migraine.

Nobody knows for certain why having migraine increases the risk of heart disease or stroke. Research in migraine genomics suggests that a number of the genes that predispose to migraine may be involved in the development of blood vessels, and it is possible that people who possess those particular genes may have subtle abnormalities in the architecture or content of the vessels that may make heart disease more likely. This is work in progress, and it is likely that we will in future come to understand the crossover between migraine and vascular disease much more completely.

Migraine with aura seems to be more common in a number of rare genetic and acquired diseases that affect the blood vessels. Examples include CADASIL or MELAS (for the former), and the antiphospholipid syndrome (for the latter). Exactly why aura is more common in these conditions is not at all understood.

Practically, therefore, whilst there is a link between migraine and heart disease and stroke, it is not something you can do anything about. All migraine sufferers should make sure that the condition is on the problem list in their GP Summary of Care Record, so that it can be factored in to any calculation of cardiovascular risk that might be done as people get older. If you are a young woman with migraine with aura contemplating contraceptive options, then it is best to avoid an oestrogen-containing contraceptive pill, especially if you are a smoker. There is no evidence, however, that similar caution needs to be applied to the use of HRT in menopausal or post-menopausal women. Otherwise, if you have migraine, it is sensible to be even more alert than you might otherwise be to the importance of those risk factors for heart disease and stroke that can be controlled. This means actually following the common sense advice that we all should follow, by not smoking, by eating healthily and exercising regularly.

Finally, while people suffering frequent migraine attacks in their twenties may experience problems with immediate and delayed memory, processing speed and spatial awareness, these are not permanent impairments. Studies of attention, language, processing speed and memory in people in their fifties and sixties show that those with a history of migraine perform equally as well as those fortunate enough not to have suffered from the condition.

What role does the neck play in causing or exacerbating headaches?

'I like a woman with a head on her shoulders. I hate necks.'
Steve Martin, 'A Wild and Crazy Guy' (1978)[28]

If you ever find yourself trapped at a party between two headache experts (and you need to ask yourself what sort of party invitations you're accepting if this ever happens) and you want to make a quick getaway, the best way to achieve this is to mention the neck, and then bid a hasty retreat. For there is really no more controversial area in headache medicine than the neck and its role in headache. At one end of the spectrum there are hugely respected headache experts who do not think that the neck plays any role in causing headache, and that in fact most neck pain is actually caused by headache processes. At the other end of the spectrum are people who believe equally fervently that the neck is the source of nearly all headaches and that physical therapy on the neck can solve the problem in the vast majority of cases. The truth, in my humble opinion, is likely to lie between these two extremes.

There is no doubt that some people's headaches are cervicogenic – that is, they arise from pain-producing structures in the neck. This most often arises from the ligaments, tendons or muscles of the neck, and for this reason cannot be seen on a scan. Occasionally one might see some trapping of the high cervical nerve roots in the neck, but the commonest points to see wear and tear on scans in the neck lie between the fifth and eighth cervical vertebrae, at which levels any nerve-trapping will cause pain and other problems in the arms, rather than higher up. The reason that pain arising from the soft tissues or the high nerve roots causes headache, rather than just neck pain, is to be found in the way that sensory signals from the neck are processed within the brain. As discussed elsewhere, this area of the brain takes inputs from the whole of the head and the neck, including at least the top three sets of nerve roots in the neck. Pain output from this area can similarly extend throughout this territory, and input from the neck can therefore cause pain experiences in the head, usually at the back of the head (the occipital region), but sometimes (perhaps particularly in people with a history of migraine) further forward.

Strictly speaking, one should not diagnose cervicogenic head-ache unless the pain is specifically brought on by touching or moving the neck. Headache arising from the neck can be a cause of people waking up in the night with head pain, as neck muscles can tighten up as they are not moved while people are asleep, but it can also present as a headache that worsens as the day goes on, as the neck muscles and other soft tissues are put under increasing strain, particularly if the neck is held in a semi-flexed position for any length of time (see the section on work triggers (page 129)).

Perhaps a more common scenario is for people to have a background tendency to a primary headache (usually migraine) and for pain and discomfort to act as a trigger or exacerbating factor for migraine. There is a vicious cycle that can be relevant here: neck pain and stiffness is quite a common feature of migraine, both as a premonitory (warning) symptom, and as a feature of the headache phase itself. People who are having a migraine do not want to move their heads very much because even simple movements can make the pain worse. Therefore, before, during and after migraine attacks, migraine sufferers may not move their head as much as they would normally do. Muscles that do not move tend to become stiff and sore. This in turn creates higher levels of abnormal sensory signals from the neck, which feed back into the bit of the brain that generates migraine, thus causing more migraines, causing more neck stiffness, causing more migraines, and so on. It is, in my experience, quite unusual for people to live with chronic migraine for many years and to escape the consequences of this on their necks.

What can be done about this? The first and simplest thing to do is to try to ensure that one does not get into that vicious cycle in the first place by keeping the neck moving. Long periods of immobility (for example, in front of laptops or smartphones) should be avoided, and if you wake up with pain in your neck or headache, you should look at your sleeping arrangements. Don't think you have to rush out and spend a fortune on a particular brand of pillow, however, as there is no convincing evidence that any specific style or make of mattress or pillow is any less likely to engender neck pain overnight than any others. As in so many things, different individuals will find different levels of support and firmness beneficial. To find one's sweet spot may require a process of experimentation, and the most expensive option may not be the best.

Beyond that, it can often be helpful to have sessions of physiotherapy directed at the neck, with the general goal of keeping the neck muscles as supple and – in most cases, with the possible exception of those who suffer from hypermobility – as mobile as possible. Finally, in a very small proportion of cases, interventions such as nerve blocks, or facet joint or epidural injections, performed by pain specialists, may be beneficial.

What is the link between headaches and hormones?

*'I am determined to have the headache Thursday, if I have
to hit myself with a rock to do it.'*
Patricia C. Wrede, *Sorcery & Cecelia* (1988)[29]

The links between headaches and hormones are complicated. There are plenty of good reasons to suspect that the
levels of hormones, particularly the female sex hormones
oestrogen and progesterone, are important for changing the
threshold at which headaches, particularly migraines, will
develop within the brain. There are several pieces of evidence that point to this: one is the tendency of migraine to
rise and fall in people's lives, and for the periods at which
migraine is most often seen to accelerate (that is, where
people are likely to have more attacks next year than they
have had this year) are those at which hormones are most
changeable, around puberty and menarche, and again in the
perimenopause. Another is the fact that, for many women,
migraines come predominantly (or in some cases exclusively)
at specific points in their menstrual cycle (most often with
or just before their periods, or at ovulation) when oestrogen
levels fall. A third is the general tendency of migraine headaches to improve as pregnancies progress, with a converse
increase in the incidence of migraine aura in the third tri-

mester, when oestrogen levels are at their highest, or when taking oestrogen-containing contraceptives.

The basic explanation for this is that high levels of oestrogen lower the threshold for the process (cortical spreading depression) that causes aura. Some women only ever experience aura when taking a combined oral contraceptive pill, or in the later stages of pregnancy. It is almost completely the opposite case for migraine headache. In this case it seems to be falling oestrogen levels that act as a powerful trigger for headache in many women. Research pioneered by Anne MacGregor and Stephen Silberstein clearly shows that, on average, women are more likely to get migraines with, or just before, their periods, and that these migraines are more severe and more difficult to treat than migraines occurring at other times in the cycle. Many women will find that they are much more susceptible to triggers such as poor sleep, alcohol and so on in the days immediately preceding their periods (of course, certain migraine triggers such as sleep disruption may themselves be features of premenstrual syndromes). Similar effects are seen in women taking combined oral contraceptive pills, usually on the second or third day following the end of their twenty-one-day course of oestrogens.

Pure menstrual migraine is one of the few varieties of migraine that can be treated pre-emptively, as it were, by taking acute migraine medication ahead of an expected attack, so long as the cycle is regular and predictable. Trials have shown that taking regular painkillers (long-acting non-steroidal anti-inflammatories, or long-acting triptans) from a couple of days before the menstrual migraine is expected, can prevent the attack from starting. Treatment is usually continued for four or five days; in 30–40 per cent of cases this will stop the attacks altogether; in some cases it will just delay or ameliorate them. Other trials show that short-term oestrogen supplementation, achieved for example by wearing an oestrogen patch from a couple of days before the period is due, can have the same effect, presumably by smoothing out the precipitous fall in oestrogen levels.

The tendency to improvement in pregnancy is presumed to be due to the presence of stable, steadily increasing oestrogen levels. This can be mimicked by taking exogenous oestrogens continuously. In the UK, taking combined contraceptive pills without any break is generally frowned upon (even though the evidence for this being in any way dangerous is sparse, at best), but most authorities will countenance the 'tricycling' regime, which usually (and slightly confusingly) involves taking four packs of twenty-one days' worth of active oestrogen-containing pills sequentially, before having a single seven-day withdrawal. The effect of this is that women will have a period (actually a withdrawal bleed, if one is being pedantic) once every three months, rather than monthly.

Whilst there are general rules of thumb about how oestrogens might affect women's migraines, not everyone's headaches have read the textbooks, and paradoxical improvement or worsening is not uncommon. The effect of hormone replacement therapy (HRT) on migraines is particularly difficult to predict. It is probably the case that for most women it makes little difference; my usual advice is to base the decision whether to commence HRT on consideration of its other benefits and risks, and to hope it will help with migraines (but also to be aware that it might make things worse).

The effect of other sex hormones is less well understood. In my experience, some women find that their headaches are very sensitive to the effect of progesterone; this can work both to improve or to worsen them. The effect of testosterone supplementation is similarly uncertain; some small trials suggest that testosterone levels may be generally low in men with chronic migraine, and that supplementation may be helpful for pre- and post-menopausal women with migraine, but more research is needed.

The same is true for the connections between headaches and non-sex hormones. Recent research suggests that having an underactive thyroid gland is more common in people with headaches, particularly migraines, but the reasons for this association are not clear. Headaches are common in people with abnormally high levels of cortisol, thyroxine or parathyroid hormone, but these conditions are fortunately very rare, and headache is rarely the most prominent feature.

As mentioned elsewhere, having migraine with aura is a small independent risk factor for stroke in young women, as is taking an oestrogen-containing contraceptive pill. This is not the case for migraine without aura. Having migraine may therefore impact on contraceptive choices. In all cases, the potential benefit of taking oestrogens (for contraception or HRT) has to be balanced against the potential risks of doing so. These are issues that should be discussed with a general practitioner or a gynaecologist.

How do you care for someone with headaches?

> *Love is a universal migraine,*
> *A bright stain on the vision*
> *Blotting out reason.*
>
> Robert Graves, 'Symptoms of Love' (1961)[30]

It is uncomfortable to watch other people in pain. In this sense, pain is contagious. It spreads from person to person. How do we react to this? Our instincts may be to comfort, or reassure. But plain reassurance is rarely enough, without explanation, reformulation and hope.

Otherwise our instinct may be to turn away, to avoid the pain of seeing others in pain. This may be particularly the case if we feel there is nothing we can do to help. In this sense the pain of a migraine sufferer is almost inevitably a private affair, rather than a public spectacle. They are quarantined. It has none of the theatricality of other forms of pain that have become commonplace in the media, in entertainment and in the works of social theorists. Scenes of violence and torture may enrapture or exhilarate, if presented in a movie or television series. There is something gripping, visceral and emotive about such scenes, so long as we are able to watch from afar, and stay separate from the need to intervene or to deal with the consequences.

This is perhaps one of the reasons why so many migraine sufferers feel abandoned. It is all very well to see someone in pain and want to help, whether you are their partner, their carer, or even their doctor. But if you do not understand what is happening (or, worse still, if you do understand what is happening but you feel that there is a degree of dissemblance), then the most common reaction is simply to walk away. Many of those who care for patients with migraine reach a point where their knowledge is insufficient and their compassion feels exhausted; many feel guilty about this, but will readily admit to this behaviour in the face of hopelessness and despair.

How do you get beyond this point, if you care for someone with headaches? The starting point in helping someone in this situation is to try to understand, as best you can, what is happening to them. The first step is incredibly simple, but not always easy: it is to listen – to properly listen – to people with headaches, and take what they say seriously. It is always good to be sympathetic, and empathetic if you can, but there are limits to this, particularly if the person you care for is suffering from very frequent or chronic headaches. Even the most caring partner can only provide so much emotional support, and it is important for those who live with headache sufferers to recognise this as well.

Then there are the practical things you can do: you can help manage the sufferer's environment, both during headache attacks and in-between times; you can be proactive in finding and providing pain relief, fluids and so on. You can help by providing a second set of ears at consultations, taking notes and asking questions; searching for information online can be difficult in the throes of a headache, and you can be the one to consult 'Dr Google', if only to make a list of questions to ask the healthcare provider at their next visit.

You can help by being strong and practical when headaches prevent the sufferers from being so. After all, it may be the headache sufferer's turn to support you tomorrow, or at some point in the future. Sometimes a physical presence is enough to provide reassurance and hope, but at other times you may need to withdraw and allow the sufferer to commune with their neurological condition on their own for a while. There are no hard and fast rules, but listening and being kind go a long way in most cases.

What does the future hold for those living with headaches?

Pain is inevitable. Suffering is optional.
Murakami Haruki, *What I Talk About*
When I Talk About Running (2007)[31]

Halfway through my medical training, I took a six-year detour, first training and then practising as an historian of medicine. If the history of medicine teaches us anything, it is humility. Doctors, it turns out, are very bad at predicting the future of their profession, or even of their small part of it. Much of what we do now may seem quaint, odd, or even downright dangerous to future generations. (Heroin for cough, or strychnine to stimulate the bowels, anyone?) Nonetheless, it is possible to prognosticate with reasonable certainty about certain trends in headache treatment.

The first is that further treatments based on blocking the effect of CGRP will make their way into clinical practice in the UK and Europe. We can be pretty certain about this because they are already in use in the USA. These drugs – the gepants – are the second generation of a drug class that has been in development since the late 1990s. The first generation went through clinical trials in the early 2000s, and were about to be released for general use in 2008 when reports appeared that patients who had continued to take them after being involved in clinical trials had developed liver failure. Unsurprisingly, the drugs were withdrawn, and several other gepants in development were also axed. However, not all gepants proved to be toxic to the liver, and in the 2010s a second generation of gepants made it safely through clinical trials (with close scrutiny of their effect on the liver function) and have made it all the way to market.

These drugs work in much the same way as the triptans do, that is, by blocking the effect of CGRP. Interestingly, unlike the triptans, they do not (yet) seem to be associated with a worsening of headaches by medication overuse, and indeed two of the gepants have been shown in trials actually to reduce the frequency of headaches if taken regularly. Rimegepant has been shown to work both as an acute treatment and as a preventive (perhaps a little more convincingly for the former). Ubrogepant has been licensed in the USA as an acute treatment, and atogepant as a preventive. A fourth drug – vazegepant – has been developed as a nasal spray, and has recently completed the clinical trial process successfully. The gepants are likely to find a place in clinical practice as acute treatments used by patients who do not respond to triptans (which may include up to 20 per cent of migraine patients), or who cannot take or tolerate them. In regard to preventive medication, they may become alternatives to monoclonal antibodies or Botox in people who do not respond to them, or perhaps those who would rather take tablets than have needles stuck in them (either by a doctor or themselves).

Other treatments that have been made available in the USA look less likely to be made available in the UK and Europe. Lasmitidan, for example, a drug that acts at a different serotonin receptor from the triptans (5-HT1F), has been licensed as an acute treatment in the USA, but will not be marketed in the UK and Europe, ostensibly for commercial reasons. This is a shame, because lasmitidan has a very favourable cardiovascular profile, and might potentially have been a good option for people with pre-existing heart disease or stroke, who cannot take triptans, CGRP monoclonal antibodies or gepants. It is to be hoped that this decision will be revisited at some point.

As lasmitidan shows, CGRP is not the only game in town when it comes to brain systems involved in headaches. Other targets are under development. One promising but arcane molecule – the pituitary adenyl cyclase activating protein (PACAP) – may have a role in migraine physiology alongside CGRP, and drugs that target the PACAP receptor have shown some positive effects in early-stage clinical trials. Whether this will make it all the way through the clinical trial process remains to be seen, of course. There is also interest in drugs that target other brain neurotransmitter systems, such as gluta-mate or the orexins. Even endocannabinoids are molecules of interest in this area. Whilst the published evidence for the use of cannabis or medicinal cannabis products in headache disorders is sparse, a proof-of-concept trial of a drug that may modulate the breakdown of anandamide (a THC-like molecule found in the nervous system) has shown some promising early results.

All of these systems are the subject of ongoing basic research in headache science. The lesson of CGRP, the triptans and the other drugs that target this molecule, is that it takes time, from appreciation that a system is important in headache physi-ology, to developing drugs that will safely and successfully target that system in the real world. However, it is unlikely to be the case that our previous method of coming by new drugs for headache – that is, purloining them from other areas of medicine – will yield much more in the way of obvious benefit going forward. The future is understanding headache processes within the brain, and finding the best possible ways of intervening in them, to make it possible for people to live with – or better still, live without – headaches.

Dr Mark Weatherall

What further resources are helpful for people with headaches, and their carers?

And I have learned now to live with it, learned when to expect it, how to outwit it, even how to regard it, when it does come, as more friend than lodger. We have reached a certain understanding, my migraine and I.

Joan Didion, *The White Album* (1979)[32]

For people with headaches there is no shortage of advice to be found online, in bookstores and in libraries. Reliable advice is perhaps in slightly shorter supply, and one should be appropriately sceptical about any book or website that promises to 'cure' headaches or migraines. As we have seen in this book, the tendency to experience headaches is part of our genetic inheritance. One can manage that. One can generally find ways of reducing the frequency, intensity and duration of headaches. One can learn to live with headaches. But they cannot, in any meaningful sense, be cured.

Excellent starting places for further information are the websites of the leading headache charities: the Migraine Trust (www.migrainetrust.org), and the Organisation for the Understanding of Cluster Headache (OUCH) (www.ouchuk. org). All the medical information on these sites has been validated by the medical trustees of these organisations, and is reliable and balanced. While you are there, if you can, why not contribute to help the extraordinarily valuable work these charities do in providing information and advocacy for headache sufferers?

NHS and NICE guidelines for the management of headaches can be found at www.nhs.uk/conditions/migraine, and www.nice.org.uk/guidance/cg150, respectively. The latter is written largely for medical practitioners, but may be of interest to those who want to understand why some treatments may be offered in NHS headache consultations, and not others.

There are a multitude of headache apps that make it easier to track headache frequency and intensity, to assess the impact of painkillers and preventive treatment, and to look for triggers. Of those, perhaps the longest-established and most widely used is Migraine Buddy, the basic version of which is free to use. Most headache clinicians will be familiar with the outputs from this and other leading apps.

Those who are interested in the history of migraine can do no better than read Katherine Foxhall's wonderful book *Migraine: A History* (Baltimore: Johns Hopkins University Press, 2019), which, amongst other things, provides a rationale for the mediaeval practice of using earthworms in plasters to treat headaches. Those fortunate enough to read French will enjoy Esther Lardreau's *La Migraine: Biographie d'une Maladie* (Paris:

Les Belles Lettres, 2015). Oliver Sacks' repeatedly republished and revised monograph *Migraine* (London: Pan Macmillan, 2023) remains, more than fifty years after it was first published, a stimulating and fascinating, if idiosyncratic, account of this condition, all the more remarkable for its first edition having been (as Sacks recounts in his autobiography *On the Move*) written in just nine days in 1968. Those wishing to understand the roots and importance of stigma as experienced in headache disorders should read Joanna Kempner's *Not Tonight: Migraine and the Politics of Gender and Health* (Chicago: University of Chicago Press, 2014).

Headache sufferers struggling with sleep might find CBT-I techniques helpful. Two books that present these are Colin Espie's *Overcoming Insomnia and Sleep Problems: A self-help guide using Cognitive Behavioural Techniques* (Little, Brown, 2nd edition 2019), and Kirstie Anderson's *How to Beat Insomnia and Sleep Problems One Step at a Time: Using evidence-based low-intensity CBT* (Robinson, 2018). These techniques are embedded in apps such as Sleepstation and Sleepio (the latter of which has been shown in peer-reviewed clinical trials to improve sleep outcomes), though these are not free to use.

Acknowledgements

Like any work based on the cumulative experience of years of clinical practice, this book owes much to the lessons I have learned from my mentors and colleagues in headache medicine, and neurology more generally. In the former camp, my especial gratitude goes to Peter Goadsby, who took the time to answer unsolicited advice-seeking emails from a junior doctor he had never met, and eventually enabled me to get a proper grounding in headache science and practice at the Institute of Neurology and the National Hospital for Neurology and Neurosurgery in London. Equally influential during my spell there was the urbane, curious and creatively disorganised clinician-scientist Holger Kaube. Holger was as different as any human being could be from Peter, and yet their opposite approaches to just about everything combined to create a vibrant, inspiring environment in which to work, learn and grow.

On the headache side, I am also grateful for everything I learned about headache from Paul Rolan in Manchester, Anish Bahra at the National Hospital and Richard Peatfield at Charing Cross. I would not have had a career in neurology without the support of Michael Donaghy, Helena Moore, Kevin Talbot and George Ebers in Oxford; Sandip Shaunak, John Ealing and Robin Corkill in Preston; Jeremy Gibbs and Tom Warner in Stevenage; and Chris Kennard, Raad Shakir, Angus Kennedy, Jenny Vaughan, Jane Pritchard, Harri Jenkins, John Janssen, Omar Malik and Michael Johnson at Ealing and Charing Cross Hospitals, as well as my many other colleagues, medical and nursing, with whom I shared patients, discussions, triumphs and frustrations.

In addition I am grateful to Lindsey Evans and the team at Headline for asking me to write this book, and for their patience while I did so. All errors, omissions and lack of clarity are entirely the author's responsibility, and not that of the team who have brought the project to fruition.

Finally, none of this would have been possible without the constant love and support of my wife, Sally, and my children, Lauren, Monty, Theo, Raph and Seb. I know, I missed that bit at medical school. But I did concentrate when it came to neurology.

Endnotes

1 Carroll, Lewis, *Alice's Adventures in Wonderland* (Macmillan, 1865)

2 Kipling, Rudyard, *Just So Stories* (Macmillan, 1902)

3 Galen, *On the Affected Parts* (2nd century CE)

4 Willis, Thomas, *Discourses of the Soul of Brutes Which Is The Vital and Sensitive Soul of Man* (Thomas Dring & John Leigh, 1672)

5 Scarry, Elaine, *The Body in Pain* (Oxford University Press, 1985)

6 Mersel, Iman, 'I Describe a Migraine' (Kenyon College, 2006)

7 Edvinsson, Lars, *Trends in Neurosciences* (Elsevier Ltd, 1985)

8 Pasten, Linda, from 'Migraine' (Poetry Foundation, 1994)

9 Harden, Holly, *On Migraines* (Michigan State University Press, 2002)

10 Carroll, Lewis, *Alice's Adventures in Wonderland* (Macmillan, 1865)

11 Gowers, William, *A Manual of Diseases of the Nervous System*, Volume II (J & A Churchill, 1886)

12 Reece, Richard, *A Practical Dictionary of Domestic Medicine* (Longman, 1808)

13 Martin, George R.R., *A Feast for Crows* (HarperCollins, 2005)

14 Franklin, Benjamin. (1736)

15 Twain, Mark, *Following the Equator* (American Publishing Co., 1897)

16 Parton, Dolly. (2021)

17 Blau, Nat. *Migraine – Clinical and Research Aspects* (Johns Hopkins University Press, 1987)

18 Editorial on 'Cluster headache' (*British Medical Journal*, 22nd November 1975)

19 Fischell, Robert, TED talk 'My Wish: Three unusual medical interventions' (2005)

20 Shakespeare, William, *Henry IV, Part II*

21 Salinger, J.D., *The Catcher in the Rye* (Little,Brown, 1951)

22 Swyler, Erika, *The Mermaid Girl: A Story* (Macmillan, 2016)

23 Judd, Naomi, Interview with *The Caregiver's Voice* (2011)

24 Sacks, Oliver, *Migraine. The Evolution of a Common Disorder* (University of California Press, 1970)

25 From *City Slickers* (1991), Directed by Ron Underwood. Screenplay by Lowell Ganz and Babaloo Mandell.

26 Auden, W.H., 'As I Walked Out One Evening', from *Another Time* (Random House, 1940)

27 Adams, Douglas, *The Hitchhiker's Guide to the Galaxy* (Weidenfeld & Nicolson, 1979)

28 Martin, Steve. 'A Wild and Crazy Guy' (1978)

29 Wrede, Patricia, C., *Sorcery & Cecelia* (Ace Books, 1988)

30 Graves, Robert, 'Symptoms of Love' *More Poems* (Cassell, 1961)

31 Haruki, Murakami, *What I Talk About When I Talk About Running* (Vintage, 2007)

32 Didion, Joan, *The White Album* (Simon and Schuster, 1979)

Index

ACE2 (angiotensin converting enzyme-2) 90–1
acupuncture 134–5
alcohol 125–6
'Alice in Wonderland Syndrome' 53
amitriptyline 85–7
anti-inflammatories 78
anti-sickness tablets 70
anticonvulsants 90
antidepressants 85–7
antiphospholipid syndrome 156
anxiety 58–9, 76, 87
aspirin 66
atenolol 88–9
atogepant 170
aura
  anxiety 58–9
  causes 34, 59–64
  dizziness and vertigo 57
  motor 53–5
  percentage experiencing 10–11
  sensory 51–3
  smell and taste 56–7
  speech 55–6
  visual 41–50
autoimmune diseases 105
autonomic nerves 13, 33

barbiturates 76
beta-blockers 87–9
body clock 13, 112, 121
Botox 96–101
brain scans 31, 142–6

CADASIL 156
caffeine 66, 121, 125, 153
calcitonin 36
calcium channel-blockers 95–6, 110–11

candesartan 89–91
cannabis 172
caring for others 166–9
cervicogenic pain 16–17, 158–60
CGRP (calcitonin gene-related peptide) 35–40, 78, 104–5, 170
CGRP monoclonal antibodies 39–40, 102–6
charities 173–4
children 150–4
chronic headaches
  causes 18–22
  diagnosis 6–7, 8–9
classification of headaches 4–5, 17
cluster headaches
  causes 33–4
  diagnosis 8
  symptoms 12–14
  treatments 77, 106–13, 116
codeine 67
coeliac disease 127–8
cognitive behavioural therapy (CBT-I) 122, 175
colds 14
consultations 139–42
contraception 152, 155–6, 163, 166
corpalgia 52
corrugator surgery 137
cortical spreading depression (CSD) 34, 63–4
Covid-19 15, 21, 90

daith piercing 136–7
dehydration 124–5
depression 76, 87
diagnosis 6–9, 141
diary keeping 72, 75, 81, 81–2, 140

dizziness 57
doubt 27
drinks 121, 124–8
drug development 38–9

endocannabinoids 78, 172
epilepsy 56, 91–4
episodic headaches 6–8
eptizenumab (Vyepti) 40, 103
erenumab (Aimovig) 40, 102–3, 105
ergotamine 61, 69
eyes 33–4

flunarizine 95–6
food 124–5, 126–8
fremanezumab (Ajovy) 40

gabapentin 94, 112
galcanezumab (Emgality) 40
gastroparesis 70
gate control theory 118
genetic inheritance 147–50
gepants 38, 113, 170–1
glutamate 148, 172

heart disease 154–7
hemiplegic migraine 53–5, 96, 147–8
heredity 147–50
history 23, 169
hormones 162–6
hypothalamus 13, 32, 33, 112, 121

ibuprofen 66, 67
illness, headaches as 22–7
imaging techniques 31
immobility, neck 130–1, 160–1
infections 14–15
influenza 14
International Classification of Headache Disorders (ICHD) 4, 5–6, 17

International Headache
Society (IHS) 4, 62

lasmitidan 171
levetiracetam 94
lifestyle modifications 119–28,
152–3
lisinopril 90
lithium 112

mAbs see CGRP monoclonal
antibodies
meals, missing 126
medication overuse 70, 71–9
MELAS 156
melatonin 112, 121, 122
menstrual cycle 162–4
microbiome 128
migraines
children 150–1
classification issues 5–6
corpalgia 52
diagnosis 7–8
hemiplegic 53–5, 96, 147–8
phases 11
symptoms 10–11
trigeminocervical complex
(TCC) 31–4
triggers 34, 120, 124–5,
162–6
vestibular 57, 96
see also aura
monoclonal antibodies (mAbs)
39–40

nausea 70
neck 15–17, 130–1, 158–61
nerve blocks 101, 110, 161
nerves
autonomic 13, 33
cervicogenic pain 16–17,
158–60
extracranial blood vessels
31–2
pain receptors 5, 29–30
neuromodulation 113–18
'new daily persistent
headache' 20–1
nocebo effect 21, 136
NSAIDs (non-steroidal anti-
inflammatories) 66, 75,
78
numbness 51, 52–3

occipital nerve 101, 110,
112–13

oestrogen 162–5
opiates 68, 70, 76
orexins 172
oxygen inhalation 108–9

PACAP receptor 172
pain
cause and effect 35
definitions 3–4, 29
gate control theory 118
referred 30–1
pain ladder (WHO) 68
pain receptors 5, 29–30
painkillers
maximum frequency 74–5
over-the-counter 66–7
overuse 71–9
paracetamol 66, 67
paroxysmal hemicrania 13
peptides 36
philosophy 23–5
photophobia 33, 131
pillows 161
pins and needles 51
pizotifen 94–5
placebo effect 135, 136, 152
primary headaches 4, 31–5
probiotics 128
propranolol 88–9
psychological therapies 83

Raynaud's phenomenon 105
rebound headaches 70, 74, 77
referred pain 30–1
remote electircal stimulation
118
resources 173–5
retina 33
rimegepant 170

secondary headaches 5,
14–15, 29–30
sensitisation, medication
overuse 78
sensory processing 29–32
serotonin 68, 95
shift-working 129
sinuses 15
sleep 112, 119–23, 153, 175
SNRIs (selective serotonin
and noradrenalin reuptake
inhibitors) 87
sodium valproate 91–4, 112
speech, migraine aura effects
55–6

sphenopalatine ganglion
(SPG) 33–4, 112–13
steroids 76–7, 101, 110
stigma 27
stroke 154–7
sumatriptan 37, 68–9
SUNA 14
SUNCT syndrome 13–14
supraorbital nerve stimulation
117–18

telmisartan 90
tension-type headaches
diagnosis 7–8
symptoms 9–10
testosterone 165
thalamus 32, 33
thyroid 165–6
topiramate 92–4, 112
transcranial magnetic
stimulation (TMS) 114
'transformed migraine' 19
treatments
acute 66–70
alternative 133–8
Botox 96–101
CGRP monoclonal
antibodies 39–40, 102–6
cluster headaches 106–13
future developments 169–72
lifestyle modifications
119–33
neuromodulation 113–18
NHS guidelines 174
preventative principles
79–84
preventative types 84–96
tricyclic antidepressants 85–7
trigeminal nerve 13, 30,
90–1, 117
trigeminocervical complex
(TCC) 16, 30, 31–2, 101
triptans 37, 38, 68–70, 109–10

ubrogepant 170

vaccinations 21
vagal nerve stimulation (VNS)
111, 116–17
vazegepant 171
verapamil 96, 110–11
vertigo 57
vestibular migraine 57, 96

women, hormones 162–5
work 129–33